Occupation-Based
Activity Analysis

Occupation-Based
Activity Analysis

HEATHER THOMAS, PhD, OTR/L
LOMA LINDA UNIVERSITY
DEPARTMENT OF OCCUPATIONAL THERAPY
SCHOOL OF ALLIED HEALTH PROFESSIONS
LOMA LINDA, CALIFORNIA

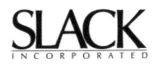

SLACK
INCORPORATED

www.slackbooks.com

ISBN: 978-1-55642-946-0

Copyright © 2012 by SLACK Incorporated

Occupation-Based Activity Analysis includes ancillary materials specifically available for faculty use. Included are PowerPoint presentations. Please visit www.efacultylounge.com to obtain access.

Heather Thomas, PhD, OTR/L has no financial or proprietary interest in the materials presented herein.

The procedures and practices described in this book should be implemented in a manner consistent with the professional standards set for the circumstances that apply in each specific situation. Every effort has been made to confirm the accuracy of the information presented and to correctly relate generally accepted practices. The authors, editor, and publisher cannot accept responsibility for errors or exclusions or for the outcome of the material presented herein. There is no expressed or implied warranty of this book or information imparted by it. Care has been taken to ensure that drug selection and dosages are in accordance with currently accepted/recommended practice. Due to continuing research, changes in government policy and regulations, and various effects of drug reactions and interactions, it is recommended that the reader carefully review all materials and literature provided for each drug, especially those that are new or not frequently used. Any review or mention of specific companies or products is not intended as an endorsement by the author or publisher.

SLACK Incorporated uses a review process to evaluate submitted material. Prior to publication, educators or clinicians provide important feedback on the content that we publish. We welcome feedback on this work.

Published by: SLACK Incorporated
        6900 Grove Road
        Thorofare, NJ 08086 USA
        Telephone: 856-848-1000
        Fax: 856-848-6091
        www.slackbooks.com

Contact SLACK Incorporated for more information about other books in this field or about the availability of our books from distributors outside the United States.

Library of Congress Cataloging-in-Publication Data

Thomas, Heather, 1971-
  Occupation-based activity analysis / Heather Thomas.
      p. ; cm.
  Includes bibliographical references and index.
  ISBN 978-1-55642-946-0 (pbk. : alk. paper) 1. Occupational therapy. 2. Sensorimotor integration--Therapeutic use. I. Title.
  [DNLM: 1. Occupational Therapy--methods. 2. Activities of Daily Living. 3. Psychomotor Performance. 4. Treatment Outcome. WB 555]
  RM735.T46 2011
  615.8'515--dc23
                              2011016450

For permission to reprint material in another publication, contact SLACK Incorporated. Authorization to photocopy items for internal, personal, or academic use is granted by SLACK Incorporated provided that the appropriate fee is paid directly to Copyright Clearance Center. Prior to photocopying items, please contact the Copyright Clearance Center at 222 Rosewood Drive, Danvers, MA 01923 USA; phone: 978-750-8400; web site: www.copyright.com; email: info@copyright.com

Printed in the United States of America.

Last digit is print number: 10 9 8 7

DEDICATION

So much of what we become is based on what we know is possible. My parents knew no limits to my future and encouraged me through all of the adventures I took on, including writing this book. Thank you for continually bugging me, "How is the book coming along?" Your guidance has brought me to where I am today.

To all of my friends and patient husband, thank you for allowing me to "disappear" for hours (and days) to write. Some of you were kind enough to allow me to follow you around with a camera, which I greatly appreciate; I know you were thinking, "She wants a picture of me doing that??"

Finally, this book is dedicated to and written with great thanks to all occupational therapy students. The future of our profession lies in your hands, and the future is bright.

CONTENTS

Occupation-Based Activity Analysis includes ancillary materials specifically available for faculty use. Included are PowerPoint presentations. Please visit www.efacultylounge.com to obtain access.

ACKNOWLEDGMENTS

It is through engagement in occupation, and watching others engage in meaningful occupations, that I have come to truly understand the complexities of what we do every day. I would like to thank those who have allowed me a window into their occupations—a brief moment into how and why activities occur. For this opportunity, I especially thank all of the clients I have served over the years. Your patience and trust have allowed me to learn about occupations beyond my own.

I would also like to acknowledge all of the faculty and staff at Loma Linda University who have supported me through this process. Thanks especially to the writing group; I never would have made it without our monthly meetings and brainstorming. You all inspire me!

ABOUT THE AUTHOR

Heather Thomas, PhD, OTR/L is Assistant Professor at Loma Linda University in Southern California. She has taught activity analysis in the occupational therapy master's degree program since 2004. After obtaining her master's degree in occupational therapy from the University of Southern California in 1998, she studied health care administration at Trident University and gained her PhD in health science in 2011. Thomas focuses her clinical work in the adult acute and acute rehabilitation settings. From 2000 to 2002, she was the Director of the Assistive Technology Center and from 2007 to 2008, she served as the Director of Occupational Therapy at Casa Colina Centers for Rehabilitation in Pomona California. She is actively involved in the Occupational Therapy Association of California, and has presented at state and American Occupational Therapy Association (AOTA) conferences. She currently serves as the California AOTA representative. Expanding occupational therapy's reach into underserved areas, she volunteers in Haiti to work with those who had been injured during an earthquake that occurred in 2010. A yoga instructor for many years, she now enjoys practicing yoga at home in Los Angeles, snow skiing, learning new occupations, and participating in social activities with friends and family.

INTRODUCTION

As a profession that uses occupations and activities as not only our goal but as a treatment medium, we must understand both the uniqueness of a client's occupations, as well as how an activity can be used therapeutically. This text is an introduction into both realms, by first explaining the process by which to peel back the layers to reveal the intricacy of an activity. It is through this deep analysis that we come to understand how rich activities can be.

It is through the process of writing this book that I have come to truly appreciate the vast difference between *activity* and *occupation*. To analyze the complexity of an occupation takes so much more depth of understanding of the person engaging in it, their environment, and the uniqueness of the occupation that they have chosen. (How true the Person, Environment, Occupation model fits as a way to understand occupation-based activity analysis!) As in an activity analysis, occupation-based analysis looks at what is required for full participation, yet goes beyond analyzing the activity; it looks at what it means for the person engaging in it and how and where it is performed for that person.

The format for activity analysis in this text follows the activity demands section of the *Occupational Therapy Practice Framework, 2nd Edition* (or *Framework*). The terminology used by the creators of this document comes from the *International Classification of Functioning, Disability, and Health* published by the World Health Organization, as well as previously published occupational therapy literature. The term *demands* sets forth this idea that activities require something from those who participate as well as requiring elements within the environment in order for the activity to occur. It is interesting that the word *demands* was chosen and not *needed* or *requested,* which are much more passive terms.

Educational standards set by the Accreditation Council for Occupational Therapy Education (ACOTE) for both master's level and occupational therapy assistant programs require that students be able to "exhibit the ability to analyze tasks relative to areas of occupation, performance skills, performance patterns, activity demands, context(s), and client factors to formulate an intervention plan" as well as "explain the meaning and dynamics of occupation and activity, including the interaction of areas of occupation, performance skills, performance patterns, activity demands, context(s), and client factors" (ACOTE, 2007, p. 656). This text is designed to help meet those standards, giving the students a firm foundation of understanding of the complexity of activity and occupation.

As a foundational skill, activity analysis is utilized throughout a student's career and on into their lives as practitioners. Over the years of teaching activity analysis, I have seen students refer back to their notes from activity analysis class to formulate answers to questions and problems posed in other classes, even in their last year of courses. Students were using these notes that defined areas of the *Framework,* using it as a reference. So, it is the hope that this text will serve as a reference for future work in occupational therapy curriculum, as it details the *Framework* and essential foundational information.

As an activity analysis text, it should be read in the order that the chapters appear in the book. Starting from Chapter 1, the reader is led through the steps of analyzing an activity. The layout of the chapters reflects the process in which activity analysis is typically completed. If one were to skip ahead to further chapters, the process may not be as clear, and aspects of the activity may not be determined.

If used as a reference text for understanding areas of the *Framework,* each chapter is designed to cover an aspect of the *Framework.* The areas of occupation that are listed in Table 1 of the *Framework* are described in Chapter 2. The body functions, part of the client factors that are part of Table 2 in the *Framework,* are explained in detail in Chapter 5. Only the body functions are explained in this chapter, as the activity demands only ask for this. Thus, values, beliefs, and spirituality have been left out. Body structures are also considered part of the client factors and are described in Chapter 6. Chapters 3 and 4 cover much of the activity demands section of the *Framework,* located in Table 3. A review of the performance skills from Table 4 of the *Framework* is discussed in Chapter 7 of the text.

To truly understand how to analyze activities, participate in the exercises and activities presented throughout the chapters. The ability to conduct analyses comes with practice, putting knowledge gained to work. While information presented in this text provides a foundation, readers will gain a broader understanding of body functions and skills as their education and experience continues.

As you read this book, I hope that you will begin to look at the world through a new lens and begin to see how a "simple" activity is not so simple—that every task has multiple factors that lead to successful participation. Our world is full of occupations that range in complexity and demand an insurmountable combination of body functions and skills. It is up to us as occupational therapy practitioners to be able to fully understand how the demands of those occupations fit with the clients and their contexts. Through this, we gain an understanding of how participation can be improved or enhanced.

Additional instructional materials are available to instructors, including PowerPoint presentations for each of the chapters. Please see the SLACK Incorporated Web site for access to these materials.

REFERENCES

Accreditation Council for Occupational Therapy Education. (2007). Accreditation standards for a Masters-degree-level educational program for the occupational therapist. *American Journal of Occupational Therapy, 61*(6), 652–661.

SECTION 1

ACTIVITY ANALYSIS

1

WHAT IS ACTIVITY ANALYSIS?

OBJECTIVES

1. Define *activity analysis*.

2. Describe the difference between occupation-based activity analysis and activity analysis.

3. Identify the current definitions of *occupations*.

4. Distinguish the differences between occupations, activities, and tasks.

5. Identify why occupational therapy (OT) practitioners utilize occupations and the goal of intervention as well as the method by which to reach those goals.

6. Describe how activity analysis is utilized by OT practitioners.

7. Explain how the *Occupational Therapy Practice Framework, 2nd Edition* (*Framework*) is utilized as a basis for understanding activity analysis.

8. Understand how the *International Classification of Functioning, Disability, and Health* and the World Health Organization (WHO) influence the *Framework*.

9. List the steps included in the activity analysis process.

The ability to analyze activities and the occupations in which people engage is fundamental to the practice of OT. Activity analysis is used throughout the OT process, allowing practitioners to understand and address the skills and external components needed for performance of the activity. *Activity analysis* is defined as the process used by OT practitioners

which "addresses the typical demands of an activity, the range of skills involved in its performance, and the various cultural meanings that might be ascribed to it" (Crepeau, Cohn, & Boyt Schell, 2003, p. 192). Occupational therapists and occupational therapy assistants (OTAs) are experts in everyday activity, not only as the end goal for their clients but in the use of activity as the means in which they will reach their goals. Thus, OT professionals learn how to look not only at activities as a whole but at their component parts and how internal and external contexts contribute to participation in the activities.

Activity analysis has its roots in the very beginning of our profession. As early as 1917, activity analysis, or *motion studies*, was introduced to OT practitioners. Principles were created and published by engineers, establishing methods in which to study the movements of workers while on the job (Gilbreth, 1911; Taylor, 1911). Following this, OT professionals began using these principles to find "what motions are possible or impossible, desirable, or undesirable; then he finds some occupation which involves those possible and desired motions" (Newton, 1919, pp. 4–5). Other professions have used these principles in their fields of practice as well, such as physical therapy, speech therapy, and engineering.

While analyzing activities may be part of the domain of other professions, OT practitioners have a unique and holistic perspective to activity analysis as a fundamental component of their practice. The OT perspective not only looks at how an activity might be typically done but how it is done and experienced by an individual, examining the internal and external influences on performance. This is what

Thomas, H. *Occupation-Based Activity Analysis* (pp. 3-11). © 2012 SLACK Incorporated

distinguishes activity analysis from occupation-based activity analysis.

For example, let's say we are going to analyze the activity of making a peanut butter and jelly sandwich. We can determine how much range of motion and strength it takes and how much sensory information is required to perform the activity as it might typically be done. However, let's say we go to Lisa's house and analyze how she makes a peanut butter and jelly sandwich for her daughter. The demands of the activity are very different. Her cupboards have child locks on them, which require the use of both hands to open. The peanut butter she uses for her daughter is extra chunky and is very thick (thus much more difficult to scoop out). Her daughter may be placing extra sensory and attention demands on her (as a 3-year-old often does). Thus, an analysis of the activity demands of Lisa making a peanut butter and jelly sandwich might be better understood as occupation-based activity analysis (Figure 1-1).

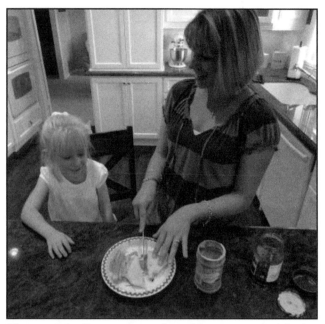

Figure 1-1. Occupation of making a sandwich for one's child.

WHAT ARE OCCUPATIONS VERSUS ACTIVITIES?

The term *occupation* can often be misunderstood and misleading. If you were to ask someone off the street, perhaps someone without a medical background, what his or her occupations are, he or she will probably begin to tell you what jobs he or she has had in the past. As a student, you may have already had the experience of trying to tell family members and friends what you will be studying and that "No, it's not about helping people get jobs." *Webster's Dictionary* (2006) defines *occupation* in several ways:

1. The principal activity in your life that you do to earn money;
2. The control of a country by military forces of a foreign power;
3. Any activity that occupies a person's attention;
4. The act of occupying or taking possession of a building.

However, medical dictionaries view a person's occupations in a much more broad, yet personal way. *Taber's Cyclopedic Medical Dictionary* defines *occupation* as follows:

> An ordinary, everyday goal-directed pursuit. Although the term is often used interchangeably with "vocation" the latter is the preferred term for paid employment (Venes, 2001, p. 653).

This definition better matches how health care professionals, including OT professionals, understand the term. The American Occupational Therapy Association (AOTA) defines occupations as follows:

> Activities ... of everyday life, named, organized, and given value and meaning by individuals and a culture. Occupation is everything people do to occupy themselves, including looking after themselves ... enjoying life ... and contributing to the social and economic fabric of their communities (Law, Polatajko, Baptiste, & Townsend, 1997, p. 32).

The term occupation *is not used to describe our profession in some countries, some using terms that stem from the ideas of ergonomics or recovery. The following are a few examples of what occupational therapy is called in other countries:*

Austria: Ergotherapeutische
Belgium: L'ergothérapeute
Finland: Toimintaterapia
India: Ergomedicine
Malaysia: Pemulihan Cara Kerja
Sweden: Arbeitsterapeuter

(World Federation of Occupational Therapy, 2009-2010)

Activity 1-1

Take a second to think about the occupations in which you engage. List 5 to 10 of them below. Then ask yourself: have each met the four criteria of an occupation as described by Carlson and Clark?

_____	_____
_____	_____
_____	_____
_____	_____

Given this definition, occupations are more than just activities; they are the activities that give our lives meaning. Many articles have been written and discussions conducted on the differences between occupations, activities, and tasks (Gray, 1998; Nelson, 1988; Pierce, 2001; Trombly, 1995). Many authors agree that occupations are a greater, more personalized definition of activities, in which smaller tasks lie (Law, et al., 1997; Trombly, 1995). Using this idea, occupations are "personalized" activities—activities that hold personal meaning and contexts for a particular person. An occupation is much more complex than an activity, which is simply looking at an activity as it is typically done, without the client in mind.

To better understand this, let's take another look at the example of the activity of making a peanut butter and jelly sandwich. An occupation-based activity analysis would more clearly show us the influence of Lisa's contexts in making the sandwich. Imagine that Lisa is a client of yours. She tells you that making lunch for her daughter is something that is important for her to be able to do. How would you analyze the activity of making lunch for her daughter? Would you examine the activity of making a peanut butter and jelly sandwich as you usually do it, or would you look at how she typically does it? Tasks can be seen as the smaller components of the greater activity or occupation, such as getting a plate out of the cupboard for the sandwich.

Activity: *Making a peanut butter and jelly sandwich*

Occupation: *Lisa making a peanut butter and jelly sandwich for her daughter at home*

Tasks: *Taking a plate out of the cupboard, getting the peanut butter out of the refrigerator, etc.*

To give further clarity to the domain of our practice of occupations, Carlson and Clark delineated how occupations are different than activities (Larson, Wood & Clark, 2003).

- There are definitive start and end points. The participant can choose to begin and to end.
- Occupations are intentionally executed and repeatable, such that something that is outside of the person's control of repeating, such as an illness or accident, are not considered occupations.
- Occupations are meaningful to the person and bring meaning to who they are as a person. This meaning may be fairly insignificant, or even unhealthy (smoking, for example), yet they still play a part in the meaning of the person's life.
- Occupations are labeled by our culture. New occupations are created every day, and the occupations people engage in change over time.

The profession of OT views occupations not only as the end goal of our interventions but also as the means by which we reach those goals. Thus, it is important to understand the depth of how much more occupations mean versus activities (Activity 1-1).

WHY OCCUPATIONS?

So we now understand that our goal is to be able to analyze the activities that bring meaning to our clients' lives, called occupations. But why do we need to analyze these occupations? We use occupations (and activities) as not only our end goal but as our means by which to meet that end goal; thus, occupations and activities are our "tools." No other profession can claim to use occupations as their therapeutic modality as we do. We use occupations or meaningful activities as intervention because we understand the greater benefit of using activities that are meaningful

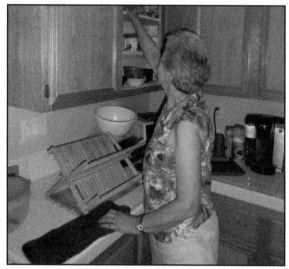

Figure 1-2. Mastery in the kitchen.

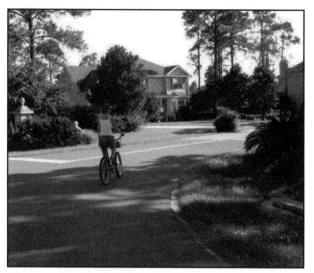

Figure 1-3. Occupations encourage greater and longer engagement.

versus other techniques or approaches. The benefits or rewards are often hidden behind the "normalcy" of everyday activities. The following are just some of the many benefits of using occupations as the center of our interventions:

+ Engaging in occupations allows clients to achieve mastery in the environment. It allows them to feel that they have some sense of control. For example, if our client Mary did overhead reaching exercises using a dowel, she may build up her shoulder strength to eventually reach into her cupboards. However, if you have her actually move cups from a lower position, up into cupboards, she will not only build up shoulder strength but also learn strategies for how she can continue to do this at home, thus gaining a sense of mastery over being able to utilize a kitchen again (Figure 1-2).

+ Engaging in occupations often results in something that the client can either see or feel. The result may be a tangible object (although many times it is not), or the result is something the client can feel. Using the example of putting cups away in the cupboard, Mary can see the results of her efforts; the cups are put away in the cupboard and she feels a sense of accomplishment. Participating in an occupation can result in a sense of accomplishment.

+ Engaging in a meaningful activity will often help the client go farther and longer toward a goal than other methods. If the attention is on the goal or the enjoyment of the process, then the client may become "engaged" and lost in participating in the activity. For example, when I go to the gym, I often will try to ride the stationary bike. In the cold,

boring gym, I can usually last about 15 minutes before calling it quits. However, if I get on my bike at home, and ride around the neighborhood, I can ride for hours. Why? The bike ride around my neighborhood is a more meaningful activity to me (Figure 1-3). I get lost and occupied in the surroundings and variety. While both are very similar and provide the same physical challenges, one will end up with a greater result, simply because it is able to get me "engaged" in it.

+ Occupations allow for greater transference toward the client's goals. Intervention that engages the client in occupations or parts of the greater occupation ensures that the intervention time will lead to application toward the end goal. For example, let's say you have your client Lance spend a great amount of time in therapy picking up beans and putting them in a cup. However, when it comes time for Lance to be able to pick up and take his own medications, there is no guarantee that the time picking up beans has helped. This is often termed *generalization.* Can the client generalize what you are doing with them during therapy time to the real world? For many clients with cognitive deficits, this is very difficult. Thus, using activities that are closer to the clients' desired occupations helps assure that they will be able to apply what they have learned or gained to their own lives.

+ Engaging in occupations requires a coordination of different skills and body systems. To help clarify this point, let's take another look at Mary's ability to put dishes away in her cupboards. One treatment strategy to help her reach the goal of putting dishes away might be to have her do upper extremity exercises. During this, she utilizes her upper body strength, range of motion, proprioception, and ability to follow directions. However, if we have her actually put cups in a cupboard, she will be working on upper body strength; range of motion; proprioception; and the skills of stabilization, reaching, coordination, manipulation, grip, handling objects, sequencing, spatial organization, and accommodation of movements. Mary is not just working on one skill or client factor in isolation but many together, learning how to use all of them together to accomplish the task.

+ By engaging in occupations, the client receives immediate feedback on performance. Feedback on performance can come from the task itself, the therapist, or from the clients themselves. For example, say Mary is trying to reach up and put a cup on a shelf. She is struggling and not quite able to reach. The therapist can give her feedback and suggestions, such as, "Step closer to the shelf," or encouragement such as, "You are almost there." But Mary is also getting visual feedback by seeing how far away she is from the goal of reaching the shelf and receives feedback from her body on how it feels to reach that high. Perhaps her shoulder is weak or feels pain when reaching. This is all feedback that is immediate and directly related to her goal.

WHY DO WE LEARN TO ANALYZE ACTIVITIES AND OCCUPATIONS?

Being able to analyze the meaningful activities (the occupations) of our clients' lives is essential to every aspect of our practice. The *Occupational Therapy Practice Framework, 2nd Edition (Framework)*, is a fundamental document published by the AOTA that describes the domain and process in which OT occurs. In this document, the OT process is described as involving evaluation, intervention, and outcomes, which are continuously occurring throughout the intervention process (AOTA, 2008). The ability to examine and analyze the activities that are of importance to the client is essential in all steps, especially in evaluation and intervention. Analyzing activities becomes instinctive and second nature to seasoned practitioners, as it is a part of understanding each client, establishing goals, creating interventions, and determining outcomes. The information from an activity analysis provides essential information:

+ Identifies needed equipment, materials, space, and time

+ Provides a knowledge base for instructing others by outlining each step and how it is done

+ Gives information on how an activity might be therapeutic and for whom

+ Helps to grade or adapt the activity to allow for greater success

+ Gives specifics for clear documentation

+ Assists in discovering how contexts influence performance of an occupation

+ Helps to select appropriate activities and find the "just right challenge"

+ Identifies areas in which the client needs help and intervention

Thus, we begin our journey with our clients by analyzing their activities by carefully looking at the details of the occupations they wish to engage in and what defines *success* in their performance of the occupation. This includes being able to analyze all of the demands of the activity for that person in his or her contexts. In order to create challenging intervention strategies, activities are analyzed to find their therapeutic benefit. The steps and requirements of the activity may be teased apart in order to adapt the activity. Before working with a client, therapists will often mentally analyze multiple activities in order to find the ideal challenge for the client during a session. The analyses often continue during the session as they watch a client struggle or succeed, and the activity may need to be adapted or graded to allow for greater challenges or successes. At the time of reevaluation or assessment of outcomes, once again the therapist must analyze the client's activities and occupations in order to establish what defines success for that client in his or her contexts. As an expert at everyday activity, activity analysis expertise is utilized throughout practice.

THE *OCCUPATIONAL THERAPY PRACTICE FRAMEWORK*, 2ND EDITION: THE BASIS FOR ACTIVITY ANALYSIS

Mentioned earlier in this chapter, the *Framework* is the basis on which this text has been developed. Therefore, it should be explained why and how this document was established. Previous to the establishment of the *Framework*, the document guiding OT terminology was the *Universal Terminology III (UT-III)*, published by AOTA in 1994. Since then, the profession has evolved and grown. Much of the language used in the UT-III was exclusively used by OT practitioners and was not recognized by other professions. A committee was developed in 1998 to begin revising this document. The committee decided that instead of revising a document that only defined terminology, they would develop a new document, which would not only establish terminology but define and clarify the domain of our professional practice. The UT-III was rescinded and a new document was created, using the WHO's *International Classification of Functioning, Disability, and Health* (ICF) as a guide.

The WHO is the leader and coordinator of global health-related issues within the United Nations. This organization directs research agendas, sets standards and norms, and studies health trends on a global level (WHO, 2001). The ICF is a document that was created by the WHO as a framework for classifying health and disability. It redefined for many what was thought of as disability, recognizing that disability has a social aspect and is not always a biological disorder but can be a result of socioeconomic or environmental factors as well. Another purpose of the ICF is to provide a common language and terminology for health professionals internationally and across multiple disciplines. This document is available publicly through the WHO Web site (www.who.int/en).

By using the terminology and classifications used in the ICF, the language used in the *Framework* is internationally recognized as well as inter-professionally recognized. The first edition of the *Framework* was created by the AOTA Commission on Practice committee and was published in 2002. The *Framework* was created as a document that would serve to "define and guide occupational therapy practice" (AOTA, 2008, p. 625). As the profession continued to grow and progress, AOTA published the second edition in 2008, with revisions that refined the original document and enriched the description of the profession's domain.

The *Framework* did more than define terminology for the profession of OT by establishing a clear definition of our domain of practice, as well as the process in which OT practice occurs. What is our focus when we work with a client? How are we different from other disciplines? If "everyday life activity" is our focus, what does that mean? The *Framework* demonstrates the complexity of everyday activities and how each component works together to allow for participation in meaningful activities. In describing the focus of practice, it also provides a foundation for activity analysis and will thus be the basis on which we analyze activities in this book.

THE ACTIVITY ANALYSIS PROCESS

1. *Activity awareness:* The first part of activity analysis is to establish what you are truly analyzing. Often activities overlap each other or become enmeshed in other occupations. Separate each activity and determine what defines success for the activity. You need to decide what type of analysis you will be conducting. There are essentially two types of activity analysis: (a) occupation-based activity analysis, which is based on a particular client and how he or she engages in the occupation in his or her contexts, or (b) activity analysis of how the activity is typically done, with no particular client in mind. Using either method, you should be able describe the activity you are analyzing in one to two sentences. For instance: "Making a cheese and onion omelet from scratch."

2. *Identify the steps required:* This is where you break down the activity into the specific steps and timing of each step. By listing the steps required of the activity, it enables the practitioner to identify the demands of the activity. This process is explained in detail in Chapter 3.

3. *Determining the activity demands:* Table 3 of the *Framework* lists all aspects of an activity that should be examined when looking at what is necessary to perform the activity (AOTA, 2008). The activity demands from the *Framework* are the basis on which this book will explain activity analysis (Table 1-1).

4. *Analysis for therapeutic intervention:* This is the step of the process in which the practitioner evaluates an activity and the needs of the client to find possible outcomes. An activity can also be analyzed in order to find ways to adapt or grade the activity to either decrease or increase the challenge for the client. This will be explained in detail in Chapter 9.

To better understand how this process works, let's take a look at a real case example (Table 1-2). Travis is a 31-year-old male who was injured on the job 2 months ago when he hit his head on a large piece of machinery and lost consciousness. He works at a factory that makes and packages potato chips. Travis works on an assembly line, putting small bags of potato chips into variety pack boxes. He has come to you to receive a return-to-work assessment. To do this, you will use your activity analysis skills, guided by the *Framework*.

Table 1-1

ACTIVITY DEMANDS

- *Objects and their properties:* The tools, materials, and equipment used in the process of carrying out the activity.

- *Space demands:* The physical environment requirements of the activity.

- *Social demands:* The social environment and cultural contexts that may be required by the activity.

- *Sequence and timing:* The process used to carry out the activity (specific steps, sequence, timing requirements).

- *Required actions:* The usual skills that would be required by any performer to carry out the activity. Sensory, perceptual, motor, praxis, emotional, cognitive, communication, and social performance skills should each be considered. The performance skills demanded by an activity will be correlated with the demands of the other activity aspects (i.e., objects, space).

- *Required body functions:* "Physiological functions of body systems (including psychological functions)" that are required to support the actions used to perform the activity (WHO, 2001, p. 10).

- *Required body structures:* "Anatomical parts of the body such as organs, limbs, and their components (that support body function)" that are required to perform the activity (WHO, 2001, p. 10).

Adapted from American Occupational Therapy Association. (2008). Occupational therapy practice framework: Domain and process, 2nd edition. *American Journal of Occupational Therapy, 62*(6), p. 638

Table 1-2

CASE EXAMPLE: TRAVIS

Step 1: Define the activity: What are we going to analyze? Decide on how you will divide the parts of his job so that you can analyze them accurately (see Chapter 2).

Step 2: List the steps of the activity: Write out the steps he must follow in order to successfully complete each activity or task. You may have several lists, one for each separate activity (see Chapter 3).

Step 3: Define the objects, properties, space, and social demands: What are the objects, materials, and equipment that he must use (see Chapter 4)?

Step 4: Define the required body functions: What mental, physical, neurological, and other body functions are utilized and challenged during the activities he must perform (see Chapter 5)?

Step 5: List the required body structures: What parts of the body are required to complete the activities (see Chapter 6)?

Step 6: Define the performance skills: What motor, praxis, sensory, emotional, cognitive, and communication/ social skill levels are needed to complete the activities (see Chapter 7)?

Step 7: Analysis for intervention: How do Travis's contexts play a role in success? How can the activity be adapted to allow for success? Are there areas that can be identified as possible outcomes for intervention (see Chapters 8 and 9)?

To begin the analysis, you ask Travis to tell you about his job and what his job entails. You then separate the different activities you will be analyzing. You define each activity, delineating what success means in each. Begin with one activity, listing each step. Evaluate what objects are needed, and what are the properties of each of these objects. Next, look at the space and social demands that

Travis has in the work setting for the activity. You will then look at the required actions of the activity. The final step is to analyze what body functions and structures are needed for him to do the activity. Using this information, you assess Travis's skills and client factors to determine if he can meet the demands of the activity. After these steps, you will be able to develop intervention plans and make recommendations for adaptations that will hopefully allow Travis to return to work.

Conclusion

The ability to analyze activities is a skill essential to the practice of OT. OT practitioners have a unique view of what activities are comprised of and what contributes to a person's participation in an activity. Our focus is not simply on activities but on meaningful activities that are part of people's lives—occupations. Occupations are the focus of our profession, not only as a goal for our clients but as the means by which we help them meet those goals. Thus, it is important to understand all of the elements that contribute to a person's ability to participate in the occupations that are meaningful to them. Using the activity demands section of the *Framework* as a basis on which to analyze occupations and activities allows the clinician to gain a full understanding of what aspects should be included in an analysis. The seven steps to activity analysis are listed in this chapter but are explained in greater detail in the chapters following, walking the reader through the process of activity analysis.

Questions

1. How are occupations different than activities?

2. In what ways are occupations used in OT practice?

3. Why do OT practitioners use occupations during intervention?

4. What does conducting an activity analysis provide for the practitioner? How does it help with the intervention process?

5. What are the basic steps of an activity analysis?

6. Read the AOTA *Framework*. Why is this document used to guide the activity analysis process?

Activities

1. Look up the ICF on the WHO Web site. How does the ICF define *disability*?

2. Interview an OT practitioner. Ask him or her how he or she utilizes activity analysis in everyday practice.

3. Create a visual representation of the steps required for activity analysis. Use a variety of objects and materials to represent this process.

References

American Occupational Therapy Association. (2008). Occupational therapy practice framework: Domain and process, 2nd edition. *American Journal of Occupational Therapy, 62*(6), 609–639.

Crepeau, E., Cohn, E., & Boyt Schell, B. A. (Eds.). (2003). *Willard & Spackman's occupational therapy* (10th ed.). Philadelphia, PA: Lippincott Williams & Wilkins.

Gilbreth, F. B. (1911). *Motion study.* New York, NY: Van Nostrand.

Gray, J. M. (1998). Putting occupation into practice: Occupation as ends, occupation as means. *American Journal of Occupational Therapy, 52,* 354–364.

Larson, E., Wood, W., & Clark, F. (2003). Occupational science: building the science and practice of occupation through an academic discipline. In E. Crepeau, E. Cohn, B. Boyt Schell, (Eds.). *Willard and Spackman's occupational therapy,* (10th ed., pp. 15–26) Philadelphia, PA: Lippincott Williams & Wilkins.

Law, M., Polatajko, H., Baptiste, W., & Townsend, E. (1997). Core concepts of occupational therapy. In E. Townsend (Ed.), *Enabling occupation: An occupational therapy perspective* (pp. 29–56). Ottawa, ON: Canadian Association of Occupational Therapists.

Nelson, D. L. (1988). Occupation: Form and function. *American Journal of Occupational Therapy, 42,* 633–642.

Newton, I. G. (1919). *Consolation house.* Clifton Springs, NY: Consolation House

Pierce, D. (2001). Untangling occupation and activity. *American Journal of Occupational Therapy, 55,* 138–146.

Taylor, F. W. (1911). *The principles of scientific management.* New York, NY: Harper & Brothers.

Trombly, C. A. (1995). Occupation, purposefulness and meaningfulness as therapeutic mechanisms [Eleanor Clark Slagle Lecture]. *American Journal of Occupational Therapy, 49,* 960–972.

Venes, D. (Ed.). (2001). *Taber's cyclopedic medical dictionary* (19th ed.). Philadelphia, PA: F.A. Davis Company.

World Federation of Occupational Therapy. (2009-2010). Definitions of occupational therapy from member countries, draft 9. Retrieved on April 12, 2010 from: http://www.wfot.org/office_files/DEFINITIONS%20-%20DRAFT9%202009-2010.pdf

World Health Organization. (2001). *International classification of functioning, disability, and health*. Geneva, Switzerland: Author.

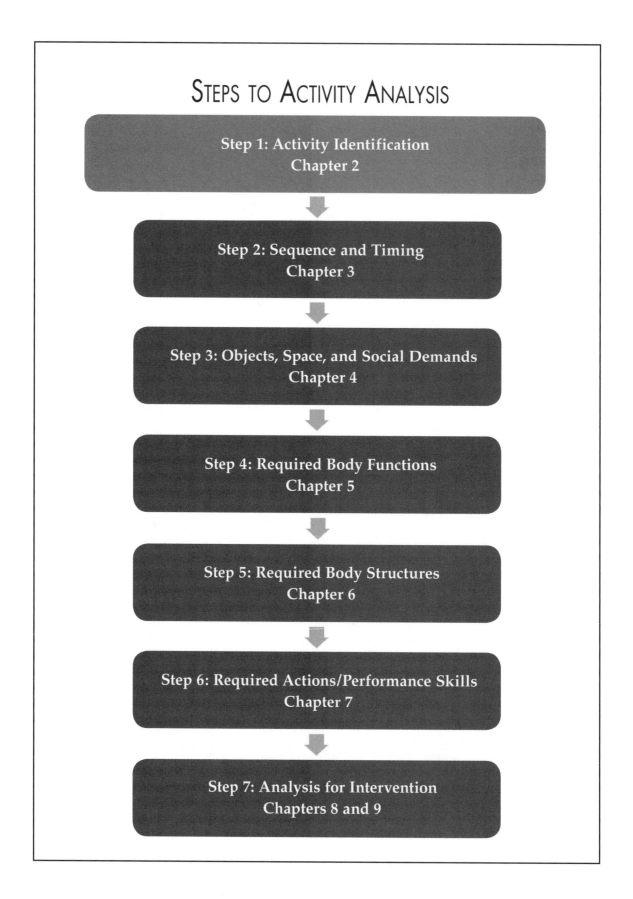

STEPS TO ACTIVITY ANALYSIS

Step 1: Activity Identification
Chapter 2

Step 2: Sequence and Timing
Chapter 3

Step 3: Objects, Space, and Social Demands
Chapter 4

Step 4: Required Body Functions
Chapter 5

Step 5: Required Body Structures
Chapter 6

Step 6: Required Actions/Performance Skills
Chapter 7

Step 7: Analysis for Intervention
Chapters 8 and 9

WHAT ARE WE ANALYZING?

OBJECTIVES

1. Determine when to conduct an occupation-based activity analysis and a standard activity analysis.

2. Understand how an occupation-based activity analysis is different from a standard activity analysis.

3. Divide a large occupation into smaller manageable activities or tasks to allow for analysis.

4. Understand why the *Occupational Therapy Practice Framework, 2nd Edition* (*Framework*) has classified and defined occupations into separate areas.

5. Define the occupations listed in the areas of occupation in the *Framework*.

6. Understand how each area of occupation relates to occupational therapy (OT) practice.

7. Identify the difference between activities of daily living (ADL), instrumental activities of daily living (IADL), sleep, work, education, play, leisure, and social participation.

8. Understand how occupations can be classified in many areas of occupation based on the client.

The first step to activity analysis is to determine what it is that you will be analyzing. As discussed in Chapter 1, there are two types of activity analysis: activity analysis and occupation-based activity analysis. The first type, activity analysis, is analyzing an activity as it is typically done, without a particular person in mind. This is helpful when looking at different activities and how they might be therapeutic. Occupation-based activity analysis is very individualized, as it looks at an activity that has meaning and contextual influences for a particular individual. Going back to the example of making a peanut butter and jelly sandwich, an activity analysis could be completed on how it is typically done, but an occupation-based activity analysis would be completed if we looked at how Lisa does it (Activity 2-1).

The first step to your analysis is to determine if you will be conducting an occupation-based activity analysis or just an activity analysis. Both are done within the process of OT evaluation and intervention. After you have determined this, you must then determine what specific activity or occupation you will be analyzing. If it is too large, it needs to be broken down into smaller activities or tasks. Some authors believe that occupations are made up of smaller "tasks" (Hagedorn, 1995, 1997). For example, if you were to look at the larger occupation of snow skiing, this occupation is made up of several activities or tasks such as putting on the gear, buying a lift ticket, getting onto the ski lift, and then skiing down the hill. Each of these contributes to participation in snow skiing and can be analyzed from an activity or occupation-based activity analysis standpoint. For many occupations and activities, breaking it down into smaller tasks is a necessary step. To decide whether or not this is necessary, think about the following:

✦ Are there more than 10 to 15 steps? If so, break the activity up into separate activities to analyze. For example, putting on pants and putting on underwear can be separated.

Thomas, H. *Occupation-Based Activity Analysis* (pp. 13-37). © 2012 SLACK Incorporated

---

Activity 2-1

WHAT ARE ACTIVITIES VERSUS OCCUPATIONS?

Using the definition of what an occupation is, given in Chapter 1 (see page 4), determine if the following would require an activity analysis or an occupation-based activity analysis:

	Activity analysis	*Occupation-based*
Putting pegs into a pegboard		
How to sew a button on a shirt		
How a client will make tea		
Riding a bike		
Mary putting dishes into her dishwasher		
Mary stacking cones on the table		
Writing a paper for an OT class		

+ Are there multiple criteria for successful completion? For example, perhaps getting dressed includes getting pants, shirt, socks, and shoes on correctly. Instead of analyzing "getting dressed" perhaps analyzing "putting on a shirt" and each other task would be more effective.

+ Are there different objects or space demands for different parts of the activity? For example, if you were to analyze "getting ready in the morning," there are parts of the activity that require the use of the bedroom (obtaining and donning clothes) as well as use of the bathroom (showering, brushing teeth). There are also very different objects required for parts of this activity. Towels, soap, and shampoo are required for showering, while a comb and toothbrush are required for the grooming part of getting ready in the morning (Figure 2-1). Finding that there are very distinct groupings of objects and settings might signal to you that the activity needs to be broken down into smaller tasks. In this example, the activity of getting ready in the morning can be broken down into tasks such as showering, brushing teeth, using the toilet, combing and styling hair, and much more (Activity 2-2).

The domain of our practice is occupations or the everyday activities that make up people's lives (American Occupational Therapy Association [AOTA], 2008). This means all activities that people may engage in are of our concern. The *Framework* helps to define what this means by listing all human activities in categories called *areas of occupation*. The most common life activities are categorized into eight areas: ADL,

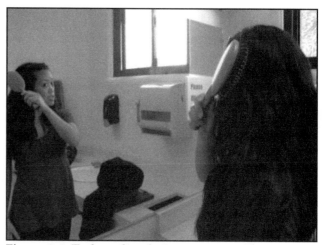

Figure 2-1. Task: styling hair.

IADL, rest and sleep, education, work, play, leisure, and social participation. Under each of these areas are categories, describing common activities for that area of occupation, followed by a list of activities that might fall under that category. For example, bathing and showering are one of the categories under the ADL area of occupation. Activities included in bathing and showering are "obtaining supplies; soaping, rinsing, and drying body parts; maintaining bathing position; and transferring to and from bathing positions" (AOTA, 2008, p. 631).

The areas of occupation are found in Table 1 of the *Framework*. They broadly define all occupations and give the reader an idea of the breadth of the scope of OT. Using this classification system helps OT practitioners in many ways.

Activity 2-2

Take a moment to think about each of the following activities. How would you break them down into smaller tasks, or would you analyze them as they are? If the activity listed cannot be broken down any further, check off the box that states "Keep as is."

	Keep As Is	Separate Activities Included In This Occupation
Washing a car		
Sewing a button on a shirt		
Cleaning the kitchen		
Making scrambled eggs		
Gardening		
Taking care of cats		

+ It clarifies the scope of our practice not only for occupational therapists and occupational therapy assistants (OTAs) but for other health care professionals and consumers. By defining all areas of occupation, everyone understands what areas we address. It exemplifies that we are more than the ADL or self-care experts but that we look at all activities that are meaningful in people's lives.

+ It is a cue for occupational therapists and OTAs as to all of the areas we are responsible for. If I was injured in a car accident and needed the services of OT, I would want the professionals working with me to recognize all areas of my life that are important. Not only is it important that I be able to dress myself and take myself to the bathroom, but it is also important that I be able to socially participate in family gatherings, engage in leisure activities, and take care of my cats. This list of occupations is often an eye-opener for students, to see the extent of what our profession entails. Yes, sexual activity and sleep are occupations that are part of our domain!

+ Each category of an area of occupation gives examples of the activities and tasks that make up that area of occupation. The complexity of everyday activities often gets overlooked. Listing the multiple tasks that are required of occupations illustrates how multifaceted some of these everyday activities are.

+ The terminology of the areas of occupation and their categories helps practitioners use universal language in their documentation. The *Framework* was created using language from the World Health Organization's *International Classification of Functioning, Disability, and Health* (WHO, 2001); thus the terminology is internationally and interprofessionally recognized. Using this language to document and discuss your client's occupations will allow for greater understanding by other health care professionals as well as funding sources.

+ Understanding what defines each area of occupation helps us determine what we need to assess and evaluate our clients. What does it mean to be independent in ADL? Using the areas of occupation as a guide, we know all of the tasks and activities this entails. If I was to watch my client Jennifer get dressed and complete her grooming independently, can I say that they she is independent in all of her ADL? What about bathing, bowel and bladder management, eating, feeding, functional mobility, personal device care, toilet hygiene, and the other activities listed as ADL in the *Framework*? Of course we must only consider all of the ADL that Jennifer considers important and a part of her life. For example, "personal device care" is a subcategory of the ADL area of occupation. This includes care and use of personal items such as hearing aids, contact lenses, glasses, orthotic or prosthetic devices, adaptive equipment, and contraceptive or sexual devices. Perhaps Jennifer does not use any personal devices. Would we consider this as part of her ADL? We would not, unless she will begin using one of these devices soon, like a prosthetic or orthotic device.

THE AREAS OF OCCUPATION

Activities of Daily Living

"Activities that are oriented toward taking care of one's own body" (AOTA, 2008, p. 631).

This area of occupation is often the first thing people think of when they think of OT. ADL are the basic self-care skills required for daily living. Christiansen and Hammecker (2001, p. 156) believe that the ADL activities are "fundamental to living in a social world; they enable basic survival and well-being." Activities such as eating and bowel and bladder management are examples of ADL activities that are essential to survival, not to mention maintaining health. These activities are often part of the routines built into our daily lives. A decline in this area is often the first sign of disease or illness (Rogers & Holm, 1994).

ADL are often called *personal activities of daily living* and for good reason; many of the activities are very personal or have to do with care of the body. For example, requiring assistance with tasks such as cleaning and wiping the body after using the toilet may be seen as embarrassing and difficult to accept. Thus, independence in these private areas of self-care often becomes a priority. As you review each of these areas, think about how important it is to you that you be able to do these things yourself.

Bathing, Showering

"Obtaining and using supplies; soaping, rising, and drying body parts; maintaining bathing position; and transferring to and from bathing positions" (AOTA, 2008, p. 631).

This defines bathing, which can be done in a tub, shower, bed, sink, or other setting, while sitting, standing, or lying down. The *Framework* does not specify that bathing or showering must be completed in a particular setting or with what equipment or objects, but it does specify the tasks that the person must complete in order to bathe the body. The first task is obtaining all supplies, including towels, soap, shampoo, or whatever the individual client requires for safe and complete cleaning of the body. The client must soap the entire body, rinse the soap off, and dry all body parts. While bathing, the client must maintain the position and move to and from bathing positions needed to clean all areas of the body. Let's go back to our client Jennifer to better understand this. Let's say she is going to bathe in a shower using a shower chair. She needs to be able to get into the shower (this can be done in many ways), sit down on the shower chair, and shift her weight and move into different positions so she can clean all areas of her body without losing her balance and falling. She also needs to be able to get out of the shower safely.

Bowel and Bladder Management

"Includes complete intentional control of bowel movements and urinary bladder and, if necessary, using equipment or agents for bladder control (Uniform Data System for Medical Rehabilitation [UDSMR], 1996, pp. III-20, III-24)" (AOTA, 2008, p. 631).

Toilet Hygiene

"Obtaining and using supplies; clothing management; maintaining toileting position; transferring to and from toileting position; cleaning body; and caring for menstrual and continence needs (including catheters, colostomies, and suppository management)" (AOTA, 2008, p. 631).

Bowel and bladder management and toilet hygiene are two areas that are often misinterpreted as being the same. The first, bowel and bladder management consists of only emptying the bowel or the bladder. This may include the use of devices or medical agents in order to complete those tasks. Examples of these are catheters, rectal stimulators, and suppositories. This category does not refer to the tasks of using and applying these aids but rather the use of them to control continence. For example, let's say Juanita has trouble with urinary incontinence. She is on a bladder program that includes self-catheterization every four hours. Her use of the schedule and the catheter to gain independence in bladder management is considered bowel and bladder management. This does not include the actual manipulation of the catheter or the use of the toilet, only her control over emptying her bladder.

Let's continue to use Juanita as an example to now define *toilet hygiene.* Juanita must transfer herself onto a commode, remove her clothing, use the catheter, dispose of the urine (and supplies as appropriate), clean herself afterwards, and transfer off of the commode in order to be independent in toilet hygiene.

Dressing

"Selecting clothing and accessories appropriate to time of day, weather, and occasion; obtaining clothing from storage area; dressing and undressing in a sequential fashion; fastening and adjusting clothing and shoes; and applying and removing personal devices, prostheses, or orthoses" (AOTA, 2008, p. 631).

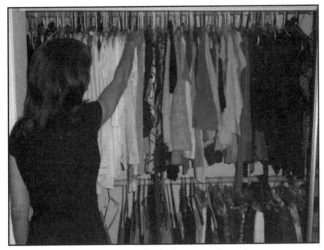

Figure 2-2. Activity of daily living: dressing.

This explains that dressing is not only about donning (putting on) and doffing (taking off) clothing. Dressing includes being able to pick out clothing that is not only appropriate for the weather but the situation the person is going to be in. Once they have chosen what they want, they also need to be able to remove it from the storage area, such as a closet (see Figure 2-2), drawer, laundry basket, etc. Once the clothing items are obtained, they need to be put on in the correct order (the underpants cannot be put on after the pants), and all zippers, ties, buttons, buckles, and Velcro (must be fastened. This applies not only to putting on clothing items but taking them off as well. Prosthetic and orthotic devices also go onto the body and are thus also included in dressing. An orthotic device, or an orthosis, is a device that is designed to control or correct a bony deformity or lack of strength or control of a part of the body (Deshaies, 2008). Hand splints, ankle supports, and back braces are examples of orthotics. Prosthetics are devices that replace a limb or body function. Examples are artificial legs, arms and hands, and hearing aids. So, while orthotics help support, control, or correct, prosthetics actually replace body functions.

Eating and Feeding

"The ability to keep and manipulate food or fluid in the mouth and swallow it; eating and swallowing are often used interchangeably (AOTA, 2007b)" (AOTA, 2008, p. 631).

"The process of [setting up, arranging, and] bringing food [or fluid] from the plate or cup to the mouth; sometimes called self-feeding (AOTA, 2007b)" (AOTA, 2008, p. 631).

The terms *eating* and *feeding* are often misunderstood and incorrectly used interchangeably. Feeding includes the tasks that occur from the plate to the mouth, and eating includes the tasks once the food reaches the mouth. It makes more sense if you think of the two in context. Imagine you are laying on a beach somewhere relaxing. Some cute man or woman (you fill in your own fantasy) is *feeding* you grapes. He or she picks the grapes off of a bunch and brings them to your mouth. You then *eat* the grapes by chewing it, moving it around your mouth, and swallowing it yourself. Thus, eating and feeding occur together but are different activities and require very different skills. A person who is right handed has a spinal injury that leaves his right side paralyzed; he may have difficulty with feeding but not eating. His ability or lack of ability to move his right hand has no influence on his ability to chew and swallow.

Functional Mobility

"Moving from one position or place to another (during performance of everyday activities), such as in-bed mobility, wheelchair mobility, transfers (wheelchair, bed, car, tub, toilet, tub/shower, chair, floor). Includes functional ambulation and transporting objects" (AOTA, 2008, p. 631).

Moving around in one's environment is essential to taking care of one's self. It is how we move from one self-care activity to another. Think about what you have done thus far today. In your sequence of self-care activities, did they all occur in one place (sitting in the tub) or did you move from place to place and into different positions to accomplish everything? In the field of OT, functional mobility does not include simply walking but moving within occupations. It includes stepping into and out of things such as a shower or car. It can also include transferring in and out of and moving a wheelchair to do self-care.

Personal Device Care

"Using, cleaning, and maintaining personal care items, such as hearing aids, contact lenses, glasses, orthotics, prosthetics, adaptive equipment, and contraceptive and sexual devices" (AOTA, 2008, p. 631).

Many people require the use of devices that assist with everyday functioning or to compensate for the loss of ability such as hearing or vision. In order to stay in working order, these devices must be cared for. For example, eyeglasses become less effective when they are dirty and have smudges across them. Taking a cleaning rag or tissue and cleaning the lenses of eyeglasses would be considered a personal device care activity (Figure 2-3). Earlier we defined orthotics and prosthetics and how donning and doffing these was considered a dressing activity. A part of personal device care, cleaning and assuring continued functioning of a prosthetic or orthotic devices, is recognized as an essential part of self-care.

Personal Hygiene and Grooming

"Obtaining and using supplies; removing body hair (use of razors, tweezers, lotions, etc.); applying and removing cosmetics; washing, drying, combing, styling, brushing, and trimming hair; caring for nails (hands and feet); caring for skin, ears, eyes, and nose; applying deodorant; cleaning mouth; brushing and flossing teeth; or removing, cleaning, and reinserting dental orthotics and prosthetics" (AOTA, 2008, p. 631).

The activities required of personal hygiene and grooming are often determined by the gender and culture of the person. Removing body hair for men may include shaving the face, the chest, or sometimes even the legs and armpits, depending on individual preference. For women, it may include the face (but not as often), eyebrows, legs, and armpits. Removal of this hair can be done in a number of ways, including using a razor (electric or manual), wax, tweezers, or lotions. Applying makeup may or may not be an important activity for women and is done in varying amounts. It is important to notice that hair washing and drying is included in this category and not bathing/showering. Trimming, filing, and painting nails is done to preference and is done to the finger- and toenails. Caring for the skin includes not only washing but looking for and cleaning any areas that may be at risk for hygiene issues. For example, those with spinal cord injuries must spend time everyday inspecting their skin for signs of pressure sores. Many diabetics must also spend extra time cleaning and caring for the skin on their feet. Occasionally using a swab, tissue, or other cleaning device to clean the ears and eyes is also essential. Blowing one's nose and removing all mucus is also an activity included in this category. Applying deodorant is often a personal choice and is often culturally guided. Keep in mind that deodorant may be applied in many areas of the body, not just in the axilla area. Brushing and care of the teeth is an activity that in North American cultures is conducted at least once a day. This includes the cleaning and application of dentures, partial dentures, or dental retainers.

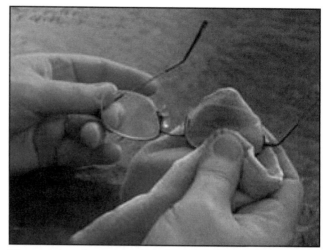

Figure 2-3. Activity of daily living: personal device care.

Sexual Activity

"Engagement in activities that result in sexual satisfaction" (AOTA, 2008, p. 631).

Sexual satisfaction can be defined in many different ways and is unique for each individual. Sexual activity does not have to involve the genitals, nor does it necessarily involve two people. The activities surrounding sexual activity are considered part of the ADL, or basic self-care, and not a leisure activity. Thus, it should be addressed as part of daily life and a fundamental part of each client's lives.

Instrumental Activities of Daily Living

"Activities that are oriented toward interacting with the environment and that are often complex—generally optional in nature (i.e., may be delegated to another) (adapted from Rogers & Holm, 1994, pp. 181–202)" (AOTA, 2008, p. 631).

The IADL are essential to living independently, however, are activities that do not necessarily need to be done by a person. For example, many men do not shop for their own food at a grocery store, and thus shopping is not an activity they engage in, just as car maintenance may not be an activity most women engage in. While delegation of many of these activities is an option, overseeing that the activities are completed and delegated to the appropriate people is in itself an activity that is part of this area of occupation.

Care of Others (Including Selecting and Supervising Caregivers)

"Arranging, supervising, or providing the care for others" (AOTA, 2008, p. 631).

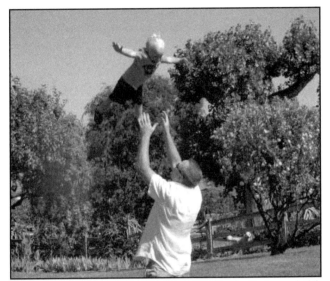

Figure 2-4. Instrumental activity of daily living: child rearing.

This includes caring for an adult family member, spouse, or friend, outside of a work setting. The care of another adult can involve providing assistance with any of the previously mentioned self-care activities. It can be as simple as administering medication twice a day or as expansive as providing total assistance with bathing, toileting, and dressing someone every day. Caregiving is not always conducted long-term but can be done on a temporary basis. This was an occupation I engaged in for a month after my 30-year-old brother had hernia surgery. He needed help cleaning his wound and with meal preparation. Other than that, he was able to care for all of his basic self-care needs. This was an occupation I was not prepared for, yet it was fulfilling and meaningful for me. Note that this category does not include the care of a child; this is explained in the next section.

Child Rearing

"Providing the care and supervision to support the developmental needs of a child" (AOTA, 2008, p. 631),

The *Framework* clarifies that caring for a child goes beyond providing basic self-care needs but also includes adequately providing the developmental needs of the child (Figure 2-4). Different theorists argue about what contributes to the proper development of a child. However, there are three general parameters to human development: biological, psychological, and social (Hinojosa, Kramer & Pratt, 1996). Many developmental theories agree that the child must be exposed to appropriate physical and social opportunities to facilitate meeting the developmental milestones typical of a growing child (Hinojosa et al., 1996) .

Child rearing also includes supervising and providing care when the primary caregiver is not available. This means finding a preschool or day care while away at work or out of the home. Not only is finding care for the child needed but also assuring that the alternative caregiver(s) meets the developmental needs of the child.

Let's say you have a client Maura, who has recently been diagnosed with depression. She has a 1.5-year-old daughter named Bethie who lives with her in her apartment. Maura feeds Bethie a bottle every 3 hours. She has not yet started her on solid foods. Bethie spends most of her day strapped into a high chair because Maura is afraid Bethie will hurt herself if she puts her on the ground. Maura spends all day watching TV and has not been out of the house in weeks. What is Maura doing to support the developmental needs of her child? Is this an area of occupation Maura is having difficulty with?

Care of Pets

"Arranging, supervising, or providing the care for pets and service animals" (AOTA, 2008, p. 631).

The task required of providing care for a pet is different for each person. There are factors that may vary the amount and types of tasks, but generally most animals require at the very least: food, water, safe shelter, and care of health needs. There may be many other tasks required, depending on the animal, the environment they live in, and the demands of the pet. For example, a horse requires a greater amount of care than perhaps a cat does (except for especially spoiled and demanding cats). Just as with the child rearing category, this includes finding and supervising the care of these pets if the primary owner is not able. So, while I am on vacation, I must arrange that someone competent and reliable can come to my home to feed and water my cats and also clean the litter box. (Finding someone to play with them for a while also assures that my sofa will not be ripped to shreds when I return.)

Communication Device Use

"Using equipment or systems such as writing equipment, telephones, typewriters, computers, communication boards, call lights, emergency systems, Braille writers, telecommunication devices for the deaf, and augmentative communication systems to send and receive information" (AOTA, 2008, p. 631).

Multiple devices are used to relay information from one person to another. Over the last few decades, our society has found greater and faster ways for us to communicate with others. Technology has begun to advance so quickly that new ways of communicating may have been developed by the time this book is printed and has reached your hands. Humans communicate using cellular, wireless, standard or land-line phones, and Internet via the use of the computer or phone. Typewriters are still occasionally used, as well as using a word processor to print out a letter. Call lights or emergency systems are used by those who are in bed, on a commode, or unable to move from a location to notify others that they need assistance. These are not only used in hospitals and medical settings but also within homes. These call lights or emergency systems are often activated by pulling a cord or pushing a button, which in turn creates a noise or flashing light to signal others.

Alternative communication devices are used by those who are unable to speak or hear. Communication boards are simple one-dimensional pieces of paper or a board with the alphabet or common words or objects on them. The user will point to or indicate which object or letter they are trying to convey to the audience. Higher-tech options are available that have voice output, speaking the word or words aloud. These devices can be activated using a number of user abilities, including movement, breath, or noise. Communication devices used for those who are hard of hearing or deaf include adaptive telephones that allow the user to receive communication via typed-in text from an operator and respond back through either speech or typing. For more information regarding these devices and the area of assistive technology please refer to *Assistive Technologies: Principles and Practice* (Cook & Hussey, 2002).

> Think about the ways you use communication devices during your day. What are the different methods you use? How much of your day includes text messaging, talking on the phone/cell phone, or checking your e-mail or Facebook account? How might you feel if you were no longer able to do these things (beyond having a break in cell phone service or your Internet service go down temporarily)?

Community Mobility

"Moving self in the community and using public or private transportation, such as driving, or accessing buses, taxi cabs, or other public transportation systems" (AOTA, 2008, p. 631).

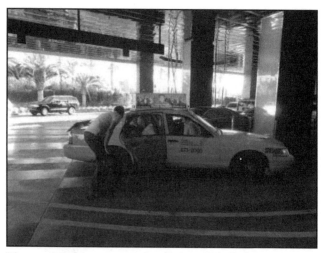

Figure 2-5. Instrumental activity of daily living: community mobility.

While mobility was discussed in the area of self-care on a more personal basis, community mobility involves the person outside of the home and into areas of the community the person is involved in. Getting to and from places such as church, school, or the grocery store is essential to many people's lives. However, independently driving is not always an option. Using a bus, taxicab, subway, or disabled transportation service are other options to allow a person to engage in this occupation (Figure 2-5). The use of each of these methods requires different tasks. For example, to use a public bus, a person must first find a schedule that indicates which bus and route will take him or her to the destination. He or she must get to the bus stop at the appropriate time, have the correct amount of money for the round trip, and be able to get onto the bus. He or she must pay the bus driver for the ride and be able to recognize when to get off the bus.

Financial Management

"Using fiscal resources, including alternate methods of financial transaction and planning and using finances with long-term and short-term goals" (AOTA, 2008, p. 631).

Taking care of personal finances is now conducted in many different ways. In the past, bills were paid using a checkbook, stamps, and envelopes. Now, many people use online bill paying services run through their banks. This eliminates the need to write out checks, and stuff and stamp envelopes. For those with physical disabilities, it has made bill paying much easier. However, financial management goes beyond just paying the bills but also includes making sure

Activity 2-3

Suzanna is an 18-year-old who is 6 months pregnant. When her parents found out she was pregnant, they kicked her out of their home, and she is now in a homeless shelter. What tasks does Suzanna have ahead of her in order to obtain housing for her and her future child?

_____   _____

_____   _____

_____   _____

_____   _____

_____   _____

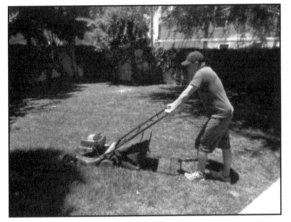

Figure 2-6. Instrumental activity of daily living: home establishment and management.

that the money available will meet the current needs, as well as help meet future needs and goals. Thus, planning and saving for the future, management of investments, alternative income or savings, and filing for income tax are also considered tasks.

Health Management and Maintenance

"Developing, managing, and maintaining routines for health and wellness promotion, such as physical fitness, nutrition, decreasing health risk behaviors, and medical routines" (AOTA, 2008, p. 631).

The level at which each person manages and maintains their health varies from person to person. Some see this as a priority and spend great amounts of time exercising and eating well. Observing and conducting any medical routines such as a diabetic checking blood sugar levels and administering insulin is part of health management. Taking vitamins or medications and applying topical medications are also tasks.

Home Establishment and Management

"Obtaining and maintaining personal and household possessions and environment (e.g., home, yard, garden, appliances, vehicles), including maintaining and repairing personal possessions (clothing and household items) and knowing how to seek help or whom to contact" (AOTA, 2008, p. 631).

Finding a place to live and keeping it safe to live in is an occupation that most people adopt as they get older and decide to live on their own (Activity 2-3). This area of occupation encompasses three major areas: (1) finding and obtaining a place to live, (2) maintaining the household environment, and (3) maintaining and repairing objects that are personal possessions. How a person defines home will define the activities required of finding a home. The activities required of a student moving out of his or her parents' home for the first time are much different than those of an elderly person who is no longer safe to stay in his or her home of 40 years and must move into a nursing home.

Once a person has established a place of residence, varying amounts of maintenance are required to keep the environment safe and up to required standards, dependent on the community. For example, some neighborhoods have requirements for lawn and exterior home upkeep, meaning the lawn must be mowed (Figure 2-6), weeds pulled, and the paint on the house kept up. For many, this upkeep is not forced by regulations but is viewed as part of the role of homeowner (or even renter). The actual tasks of maintaining the exterior home environment (mowing the lawn, pulling weeds, etc.) do not necessarily need to be done by the person but are arranged to be completed by someone else. Thus, part of this area of occupation is finding help for these tasks (i.e., calling a gardener or hiring the teenager next door to mow the lawn).

Maintenance of a home also includes assuring that the interior is kept in repair and safe. Thus, cleaning, mopping, vacuuming, dusting, and picking up trash are a few of the activities included as part of this area of occupation. While people engage in varying degrees of this occupation (and enjoy it in even greater degrees of variation), it is still essential to living in a healthy environment. Also, part of this area of occupation is the concept of maintaining or repairing possessions. This can include clothing (laundering and storing), automobiles, appliances, and all objects within the home.

For all of the activities in this area of occupation, the person does not have to do the actual maintenance or repair but simply know when and how to address it and obtain assistance when needed. Even in a small studio apartment, one needs to know what to do when a light bulb burns out or the hot water stops working.

A person's ability to maintain his or her home environment is often one of the first occupations to deteriorate with the onset of an illness or the progression of a disease. Limitations can be caused by not only physical limitations but by cognitive or mental health illnesses. For example, Nancy and Bob have been married for 56 years. Both of them have shared the activities encompassing home maintenance, each taking responsibility for different aspects. While Bob assured that the yard was always well groomed, the peach trees trimmed, snow shoveled from the driveway, and appliances in working order, Nancy took care of the interior of the home, doing the family laundry and keeping the bathrooms and living areas clean. Nancy was diagnosed with Alzheimer's disease 4 years ago. As the disease progressed, Bob found that Nancy was leaving many of the cleaning tasks uncompleted or undone. Dust began to build on the bookshelves, and dog hair began to build up so thick on the couch, it looked a different color. Bob walked into the basement one day to find the floor covered in soap bubbles. Mary had mistakenly put dish soap into the clothes washing machine. Although Nancy had completed these occupations for so many years, Bob decided to have a housekeeper come once a week to help complete some of the activities Nancy was struggling with. Bob assured that his home was maintained and cared for by recognizing what was needed in order to be safe and contacted someone for assistance.

Meal Preparation and Cleanup

"Planning, preparing, serving well-balanced, nutritional meals and cleaning up food and utensils after meals" (AOTA, 2008, p. 631).

Much like home maintenance and repair, meal preparation is done in varying degrees by different people. Meal preparation begins with the process of deciding what to prepare and what items and ingredients are needed. Interestingly, this area of occupation is defined as concerning only "well-balanced, nutritional meals." For many (especially busy students?), meal preparation entails obtaining nourishment in forms that would not be considered well balanced. Nonetheless, meal preparation, or cooking, is done in a variety of ways. Meal preparation includes not only the preparation of food but serving it on the appropriate dish, bowl, or platter. For example, cooking soup is only complete when it is poured into bowls. At the completion of preparing the meal is cleaning up all materials and objects that were used in the process. This includes washing all dishes and utensils, putting away any unused food, and wiping up surfaces that were used. While some of the tasks included here sound much like the cleaning tasks included under "home management," because this may occur during the process of preparing a meal, or is done in conjunction with the completion, it is considered as part of this occupation. Not included in this occupation is the activity of eating and feeding. The process of creating food for consumption does not include the person eating it. You may encounter clients who enjoy the occupation of meal preparation but not eating or vice versa.

Religious Observance

"Participating in religion, an organized system of beliefs, practices, rituals, and symbols designed to facilitate closeness to the sacred or transcendent" (Moreira-Almeida & Koenig, 2006, p. 844).

Religious occupations are those activities surrounding involvement in organized rituals or practices that are used to demonstrate beliefs (Billock, 2009). The terms *spirituality* and *religion* are often misinterpreted as meaning the same. While inter-related, spirituality is an internal experience, a "personal quest for understanding answers to ultimate questions about life, about meaning, and the sacred" (AOTA, 2008; Moyers & Dale, 2007, p. 28). Spirituality is not an activity or occupation but occurs within the person as a result of engagement in occupations. Religion is used as a way to reach into the spiritual aspects of the self; however, spiritual experiences do not necessarily need to occur during religious occupations (Billock, 2009). It is often through the religious occupations that many hope to reach a greater understanding of the spiritual self and a sense of something greater than themselves.

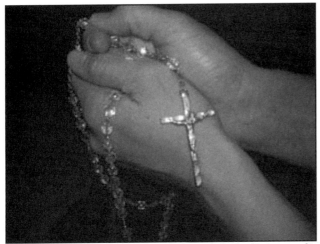

Figure 2-7. Instrumental activity of daily living: religious observance of praying with a rosary.

There are thousands of organized religions, each with their own set of rituals and practices. For some, there are weekly meetings or church services. It is during these meetings that there are actions and behaviors expected of those attending. In some church services, there is singing, reading, listening to a sermon, and reading verses or incantations aloud. Physical actions such as kneeling or moving through a series of motions a certain number of times is required. A very common physical activity for Catholics is holding a rosary, which is a cross on a string of 59 beads (Figure 2-7). The string of beads is held and manipulated as a prayer is said for each bead. Other religious activities include attending classes, going to confession, praying, and reading the Bible or other reading material. There are some religions that utilize animal sacrifice as part of their rituals.

Safety Procedures and Emergency Maintenance

"Knowing and performing preventive procedures to maintain a safe environment as well as recognizing sudden, unexpected hazardous situations and initiating emergency action to reduce the threat to health and safety" (AOTA, 2008, p. 631).

The activities that comprise this type of occupation are either ongoing preventative measures or immediate reactions to emergency situations. Ongoing preventative measures are taken to ensure that the environments that the person is in are safe from immediate or eventual danger. It requires that the person understand threats to safety and how to prevent them. For example, a person must know that he or she must not set newspaper on top of a stove. Safety procedures are often incorporated within other occupations, such as meal preparation.

Shopping

"Preparing shopping lists (grocery and other); selecting and purchasing items; selecting method of payment; and completing money transactions" (AOTA, 2008, p. 631).

Purchasing items and the activities that lead up to the purchase are what allows for providing the items needed for survival such as food, water, and clothing. It is also a form of leisure and enjoyment for many people, where items are purchased for other reasons other than for survival. For example, Carey wants to purchase a new video game. This is not necessary for Carey's survival (although he may try to convince his wife otherwise). In order to purchase the game, he will need to find a place where it is sold. There are multiple ways shopping can occur: in a store, online, from a catalog, from a salesperson, via phone, from a personal ad (either placed in a newspaper or online), from a yard sale, or at an outdoor market. Let's say Carey decides to purchase the video game online. He would need to look at the prices from different vendors to find the lowest price. He would need to choose a method of payment, which is usually via credit card when purchasing online. Completing the purchase would require providing the appropriate credit card and shipping information. If Carey was not able to purchase the game online, he might chose to go to a store. If so, he would need to navigate within the store in order to find the game he is looking for. He would take the game to a checkout counter and pay the attendant with cash, credit, or a check. However, having an attendant at the checkout counter is optional at some stores, as self-checkout machines are becoming more common in larger department stores. This would require Carey to scan in the game and follow the directions on a screen to provide payment.

Rest and Sleep

"Includes activities related to obtaining restorative rest and sleep that supports healthy active engagement in other areas of occupation" (AOTA, 2008, p. 632).

Rest

"Quiet and effortless actions that interrupt physical and mental activity resulting in a relaxed state (Nurit & Michel, 2003, p. 227). Includes identifying the need to relax; reducing involvement in taxing physical, mental, or social activities; and engaging in relaxation or other endeavors that restore energy, calm, and renewed interest in engagement" (AOTA, 2008, p. 632).

Humans require periods of inactivity within their day in order to function (Figure 2-8). By resting, we allow our bodies to regain energy to re-engage in activities. Physical and mental activity can be taxing over a period of time. The amount of rest required is often greater in some people more than others, such as with those recovering from an illness and with decreased physical, cognitive, or aerobic capacity. Physical rest occurs by allowing muscle tension to reduce and the amount of muscle contractions to decrease. For example, if standing for long periods, a rest may include sitting or lying down. Mental rest occurs by allowing little to no mental processing of information or problem solving. People choose to engage in this occupation in many ways. For many Americans, watching television is the favored way to rest. Watching television allows for passive engagement in an activity that utilizes only sensory processing of what is seen and heard. The body is allowed to be inactive while cognitive abilities are minimally challenged. For some, television is not considered rest or relaxing. For those people, greater quiet and relaxation are required in order to fully allow the mind and body to rest. Meditation and visual imagery are examples of activities some people use to engage in rest.

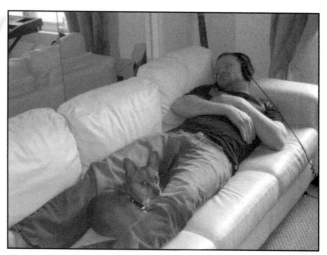

Figure 2-8. Rest and sleep.

Sleep

"A series of activities resulting in going to sleep, staying asleep, and ensuring health and safety through participation in sleep involving engagement with the physical and social environments" (AOTA, 2008, p. 632).

Since the genesis of the profession, OT as a profession has professed the importance of a balance of work, rest, and play. However, it was not until the second edition of the *Framework* that sleep was identified as an occupation and thus part of OT's domain. Sleep science studies have identified the value that sleep has on physical and mental health (McKnight-Eily et al., 2008). Although it is an occupation that is so essential to well-being, the role of OT in sleep is just beginning to emerge (West, 2009).

While engaged in sleep, the body and mind are at rest, with eyes closed, and there is little to no responsiveness to the external environment. It is during sleep that the brain changes into cycles of brain-wave activity, with periods of dreaming. It is disengagement from the external environment that begins the process of allowing the mind and body to be at rest. To allow the mind to become unconscious, one must allow the brain to release control over staying alert to internal and external stimuli (*Mosby's Dictionary*, 2006). Engagement in a sleep state might be impaired by internal stimuli such as pain, in which the brain continues to process information from the body. Internal stimuli that distracts the mind from engagement in sleep is continuous through processing. In order for this occupation to be successful, both the body and mind must disengage from activity.

Sleep Preparation

"(1) Engaging in routines that prepare the self for a comfortable rest, such as grooming and undressing, reading or listening to music to fall asleep, saying goodnight to others, and meditation or prayers; determining the time of day and length of time desired for sleeping or the time needed to wake; and establishing sleep patterns that support growth and health (patterns are often personally and culturally determined)" (AOTA, 2008, p. 632).

The activities leading up to engagement in sleep have been divided into two separate categories. The first category is related to preparing body and mind for the occupation of sleep, and the second is related to preparing the environment. Preparing the body includes activities such as removing clothes worn during the rest of the day and donning sleepwear, brushing teeth, and washing the face or body. These activities are performed in order to facilitate a more restful experience. For example, changing out of the clothes that were worn all day allows the body to be relieved of any uncomfortable sensory input and thus allow for a deeper and more comfortable sleep. Many of these activities become part of a daily pattern and are routine, with the same activities occurring every day prior to going to sleep.

The mind is prepared for sleep by engaging in relaxing activities that allow thought patterns to slow and retreat. The slowing of our thought processes

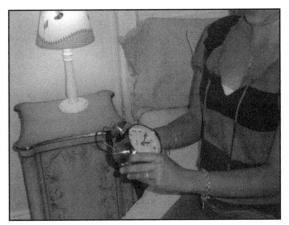

Figure 2-9. Rest and sleep: sleep preparation.

occurs as we relax and approach a state of sleep. How one reaches this relaxed state varies according to personal beliefs and values. It is also dependent upon how well the person is able to calm the mind to the point of giving up consciousness. Some people require a time period of quiet activity such as reading or listening to music before retiring to sleep. Another technique utilized is meditation or visualization.

Consciously deciding to go to sleep is also part of the mental processes required of sleep preparation. Choosing when to sleep and wake allows for establishment of sleep/wake cycles that are healthy and provide adequate opportunity for the body to rejuvenate. This occurs with an average of 6 to 8 hours of continuous sleep. To take place, one must plan what time from during the 24-hour period will allow for this (Figure 2-9). If a person must be awake at 7 a.m., he or she must prepare to be asleep by 11 p.m. to get 8 hours of sleep. Mentally processing this is an activity that is part of the preparations for healthy sleep. For people with the inability to schedule 6 to 8 hours of sleep, scheduling sleep may be more difficult. This is the case in those who work in jobs that demand long shifts and scattered windows of time in which to sleep. Crab fishermen often work 24- to 30-hour shifts with little to no sleep and must schedule intermittent nap periods while the boat travels from one fishing spot to another.

"(2) Preparing the physical environment for periods of unconsciousness, such as making the bed or space on which to sleep; ensuring warmth/coolness and protection; setting an alarm clock; securing the home, such as locking doors or closing windows or curtains; and turning off electronics or lights" (AOTA, 2008, p. 632).

Assuring a comfortable and secure environment facilitates the ability to engage in sleep and stay asleep. This requires reducing the amount of sensory stimuli during time in which sleep occurs. Limiting the amount of light in the area may require closing window blinds or doorways and shutting off lights. Removing other arousing stimuli from the environment (or removing the person from the stimulating environment) will also allow for greater ability to engage in sleep. For example, for a person trying to sleep, a crying puppy would be a distraction from full engagement in sleep. Other aspects of the environment, such as thermal regulation, modifying how much the body will be exposed to heat or cold during sleep, involves adjusting and setting any environmental heating or cooling equipment as well as providing appropriate covering for the body while sleeping. Most important of all of the physical preparations is finding a place to lay the body, such as on a bed or other surface. For most people, this means pulling back the covers and sheets on a bed to allow enough space to lay down and then pulling the covers back up and over their bodies.

Sleep Participation

"Taking care of personal need for sleep such as cessation of activities to ensure onset of sleep, napping, dreaming, sustaining a sleep state without disruption, and nighttime care of toileting needs or hydration. Negotiating the needs and requirement of others within the social environment. Interacting with those sharing the sleeping space such as children or partners, providing nighttime care giving such as breastfeeding, and monitoring the comfort and safety of others such as the family while sleeping" (AOTA, 2008, p. 632).

The actual participation in sleep includes ensuring that there is adequate engagement in the activity and allowing for necessary actions while sleeping. While engaging in sleep, as humans we move, interact with others, and respond appropriately to external stimuli as needed. For example, once we are immersed in sleep (see definition above), we unconsciously regulate our activities and responses to assure continuation of sleep cycles. For example, we may turn our bodies in our sleep when we sense discomfort. We may put an arm or leg around the person sleeping next to us or even pull up the covers, without ever becoming fully conscious. We may disrupt sleep to get up and use the bathroom. Upon certain sounds or sensations, we alert ourselves to action to become fully alert (such as hearing a baby cry or an alarm go off).

Education

"Includes activities needed for being a student and participating in a learning environment" (AOTA, 2008, p. 632).

Formal Educational Participation

"Including the categories of academic (e.g., math, reading, working on a degree), nonacademic (e.g., recess, lunchroom, hallway), extracurricular (e.g., sports, band, cheerleading, dances), and vocational (prevocational and vocational) participation" (AOTA, 2008, p. 632).

The activities that encompass attending an educational program or school include not only the academic aspects of learning and participation but also the out-of-classroom activities such as recess and mealtimes. Activities that may occur outside of class time such as being part of a school band, being on a school sports team, and attending school functions such as a dance or event are all part of being a student. It is through all of these activities that students learn about the world and how to interact with those around them. Some educational programs provide training for certain jobs or professions, and may include on-the-job training or internships.

Samantha is 5 years old and just started kindergarten. She found that the activities that occur during kindergarten are much different than what was happening at home. She starts her day by getting on the school bus that picks her up at the end of her block. She must patiently wait for the bus and board in an orderly fashion. She must find a seat and sit in the seat while the bus transports her to school, making a few stops on the way to pick up other students. When at school, she must find her classroom and put her backpack at her desk. She must listen for when the bell rings, which means it is time for class to start. She participates in many activities during the class time, learning how to write letters and how to share with others. When she needs to use the restroom, she must ask the teacher for permission. She takes herself to the bathroom and comes back to the classroom when finished. At snack time, she goes to the cafeteria where she must pick up a container of milk or juice and one cracker. During recess, she plays with other children, learning how to interact and share equipment and toys. When the day is over, she gets back on the bus and must exit the bus at the same point she got on, at the end of her block. All of these activities are part of her participation in formal education.

> List all of the activities that you currently participate in as an OT student.

Exploration of Informal Personal Educational Needs or Interest (Beyond Formal Education)

"Identifying topics and methods for obtaining topic-related information or skills" (AOTA, 2008, p. 632)

Obtaining education outside of a formal setting occurs in many different venues and ways. If knowledge is needed in a particular area, the specific topics must be identified in order to determine methods in which they may be learned. For example, Jean is an occupational therapist who has decided she would like to travel to Haiti to work as a volunteer occupational therapist. In order to fully understand what she needs to know before she goes, she contacts another occupational therapist who has already traveled and worked there. She finds that she needs to be prepared to speak basic Haitian Creole, the native language spoken. Jean does an Internet search for Haitian Creole lessons and finds a podcast series to download. All of these activities were in preparation for the informal education she hopes to engage in. Exploring the different methods in which to gain information is much more extensive, and yet much easier in many ways, now that so much information is posted on the World Wide Web. A Web search can provide information on topics, what educational needs there are for a specific topic, and where to gain further information. A search on one topic may lead to ideas for other topics. Searching the Web is only one way to explore informal education. Talking to others, calling organizations, and reading the newspaper are all examples of how informal education topics can be researched and discovered.

Informal Personal Education Participation

"Participating in classes, programs, and activities that provide instruction/training in identified areas of interest" (AOTA, 2008, p. 632)

The ways in which we are able to engage in learning have evolved over the years to allow for the acquisition of knowledge to occur almost anywhere.

As with the aforementioned example of Jean, she was able to learn basic Creole while on her hour-long commute every day, listening to the lessons on her MP3 player. Informal education occurs in classrooms, homes, street corners, and senior centers, just to name a few. Learning a new activity, skill, or knowledge can occur independently of others, by engaging in activities that encourage learning such as reading, listening to audio information, or learning through engagement in the activity and learning through trial. Participation in informal education can occur in conjunction with or guided by others. Classes or instruction may be led by a teacher or guided by students with greater experience.

Informal education includes gaining skill or knowledge that is not part of a formal educational program. Interests outside of formal educational can include leisure, social, or health-related topics. Yoga, kickboxing, painting, and English as a second language classes are all examples of informal education. It includes not only the classes but also the activities that facilitate the learning process. For example, Jill is 38 years old and has always wanted to learn how to play the piano. She began taking weekly piano lessons from a neighbor. Her engagement in this learning was not limited to those weekly lessons but also included her daily practice on the piano. After 6 months of lessons, she performed in her first recital, able to play one of her daughter's favorite songs.

> What informal education activities have you engaged in?

Work

"Includes activities needed for engaging in remunerative employment or volunteer activities" (Mosey, 1996, p. 341).

Employment Interests and Pursuits

"Identifying and selecting work opportunities based on personal assets, limitations, likes, and dislikes relative to work" (adapted from Mosey, 1996, p. 342).

How did you decide to become an occupational therapist or OTA? Did you look for jobs that addressed your strengths and weaknesses? Did you talk to others who are in the field? Perhaps you found out about OT through personal experience. Once you decided that this was the profession you wanted to get into, how did you find about the requirements for practice? Identifying work options involves finding work or career opportunities that match personality traits and desires. Finding out about a career can occur spontaneously or by chance such as when listening to the radio, watching TV, or encountering the profession through live experiences. Exploring career options can also occur through deliberate investigation by taking competency and job matching assessments. Some people go through job counseling with a career counselor to find the right match for them.

Once an area of work is identified, pursuing that career or job requires searching and identifying job opportunities that are available. This is done in many ways, including searching the Internet, reading the newspaper, looking at job postings, and talking to human resources or recruiting departments. Pursuing a particular job may require personally speaking to someone from companies that the person wishes to work for, as not all job opportunities are posted or readily available to the public.

Employment Seeking and Acquisition

"Identifying job opportunities, completing and submitting appropriate application materials, preparing for interviews, participating in interviews and following up afterward, discussing job benefits, and finalizing negotiations" (AOTA, 2008, p. 632).

Obtaining employment once a job opportunity has been identified involves a number of common activities that are required for most jobs. Of course, each job opening may have different requirements of the applicant, so the first step to seeking out employment for a particular opening would be to ascertain what is required to apply for the job. Most employers require an employment application to be completed, either by pen and paper or on the Internet. The application must be submitted to the appropriate department or employee. Along with the application, some employers require other materials to be submitted such as a résumé, background check, or sample work. After the application is accepted, the next step may be an interview, which can occur in person, over the phone, or via the Internet. The applicant prepares for this interview by gathering information regarding the company and job position and by thinking about how he or she might answer questions during the interview. The appropriate clothing must be selected for the interview if it will occur in person or via a Webcam. For some jobs openings, there is a series of interviews that take place, with some interviews taking place as a group, where multiple applicants are interviewed at the same time. Testing or competency assessments are part of some job application processes, which precede or follow the interview.

Job Performance

"Including work habits, for example, attendance, punctuality, appropriate relationships with coworkers and supervisors, completion of assigned work, and compliance with the norms of the work setting" (adapted from Mosey, 1996, p. 342).

Once employment is obtained, to remain employed requires that performance meet the expectations of the employer. This means the employee must maintain regular work habits of coming to work and leaving on time and being productive in the assigned job duties while at work. For each job these expectations will be different, according to the type of work, the setting, and the employer's expectations. There are some employers who do not expect employees to arrive at a certain time every day but have high expectations of employee productivity once they are at work. These employers believe in quality and quantity of work, not the number of hours it takes to get the work done. However, this does not work in every setting, and for most Western jobs, specific hours are determined for employees. Job performance may require engaging in activities involving a variety of skills, including motor movements, cognitive processing, and social interaction. Social interaction may occur between the employee and customers, with others in the community, or with other employees (not to mention the employer and supervisors). The expectation for social interaction varies according to the amount the employee is required to interact with others, as well as the culture of the environment. In some settings, use of foul language and yelling are appropriate, while in others the use of certain terms would be grounds for termination. The activities and level of skill needed are dependent on the type of job and the expectations of the employer. The employee must understand these expectations and meet them in order to maintain employment in that position.

Retirement Preparation and Adjustment

"Determining aptitudes, developing interest and skills, and selecting appropriate avocational pursuits" (AOTA, 2008, p. 632).

Retirement is voluntary discontinuation of employment, or complete cessation of work, which typically occurs at the age of 65 or older. For many people, work provides a sense of efficacy, an avenue for socialization, and self-esteem (McMinn, 2009).

Without activities to replace these needs, many retired people decline in physical and mental health (Dave, Rashad, & Spasojevic, 2008). Depression is very common in those who retire, and they do not find adequate avenues in which to fulfill the needs that were met through work.

Filling the void that is left by retirement can be done in many ways. This time that is now not obligated toward work is seen by many as a time to engage in those activities that they did not have time for while working full time, such as traveling, participating in leisure activities, or volunteering for philanthropic organizations or causes. Healthy transition from the role of worker to retiree requires preplanning—setting future goals and desires for what occupations and roles will meet intrinsic needs. Socioeconomic status plays a large role in these plans, as income stream shifts from receiving a paycheck, to social security payments and any retirement funds the person had set aside. Many retirees have difficulty meeting expenses with the extreme cut in income, with some entering into poverty. Physical health may limit retirement adjustment if mobility, pain, or physical weaknesses restrict the ability to engage in desired occupations.

Community resources and access to environments that lend themselves to productive retirement also influence adjustment to this role shift. For those in rural areas, there is limited access to community activities, and public transportation outside of the home may be restricted. However, even without access to community, activities around the home can fill the day with meaning. For example, Mildred was a full-time elementary school teacher in a small farm town. She and her husband live on 500 acres of farm land, 20 miles from town. Now that she and her husband are retired, they love to go fishing at the local lake, camping in their RV, and spending time with their grandchildren. Mildred has a garden that requires constant attention during the spring and summer months, always has a quilt or blanket she is making (Figure 2-10), and has started her own line of underwear and tops, which she sells at the local market. Mildred states, "I am busier now than when I was working."

The example of Mildred is one end of the spectrum of retirement adjustment, while at the other lie those who do little with the time they now have. For these people, they had little planned for retirement or have little desire to engage in anything other than rest. Ernie is Mildred's former employer, who lives a few miles down the road. At Ernie's retirement party, he told Mildred, "All I am going to do when I retire is sit and rock in my rocking chair." For 3 years now, that is what Ernie has done every day; he sits in his rocking

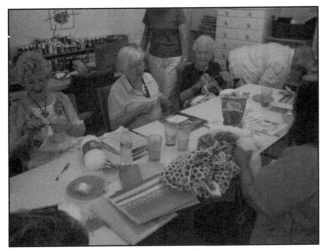

Figure 2-10. Work: retirement adjustment.

chair and watches television. Ernie's plan for transition from the role of principal of an elementary school to retiree did not include replacing the intrinsic rewards he gained from work and was a choice he made without awareness of difficulties he may encounter in adjusting to this new role. Common to many retirees, adjusting to the absence of the worker role can cause a decline in physical and mental health.

Planning for retirement requires looking for new roles and occupations that provide enriching experiences to help support health. This includes matching one's strengths and abilities to opportunities that align with the person's interests. Retirement can also be a time in which skills can be gained or knowledge sought. An assessment of life goals, what a person hopes to have accomplished in life, can lead to finding those meaningful occupations to pursue during the retirement years. Re-exploring past occupations and interests, such as ones engaged in earlier in life, is often part of successful retirement planning. OT practitioners address these occupations with clients who may be entering into this stage of life by using assessments that evaluate interests and abilities and matching these up to possible occupations. Constructing a "productive day" schedule, which gives the retiree a routine and tasks to do throughout the week, can be created with the client. These are just a few examples of how OT plays a role in retirement planning, but are also how a person can engage in this occupation on his or her own to assure healthy adjustment to retirement.

Volunteer Exploration

"Determining community causes, organizations, or opportunities for unpaid 'work' in relationship to personal skills, interest, location, and time available" (AOTA, 2008, p. 632).

Prior to engagement in volunteerism, the potential volunteer must explore the different types of philanthropic work available and determine what he or she deems as worth contributing time to. Volunteer work is often done in efforts to increase the well-being of mankind or improve conditions of what one believes to be an issue or charity in need. Skills offered by volunteers range from stuffing envelopes and making phone calls to being a board member of a nonprofit hospital or serving as a physician in a Third World country. Finding opportunities for volunteerism can occur through active or passive mechanisms. Active pursuit of volunteer opportunities occurs when the potential volunteer seeks out volunteer organizations and opportunities based on his or her skill set and time he or she is willing to contribute. For example, a person may decide that he or she wants to work with underprivileged or at-risk youth and contact the local high school or Boys and Girls Club. Volunteer opportunities also present themselves in the communities or organizations in which potential volunteers already participate in. For example, a mother may be asked to serve in her daughter's Girl Scout troop. As a passively presented volunteer opportunity, the mother would then explore this volunteer opportunity to determine if it would be a good fit with her skills and time available.

Volunteer Participation

"Performing unpaid 'work' activities for the benefit of identified selected causes, organizations, or facilities" (AOTA, 2008, p. 632).

Once a volunteer opportunity has been explored and identified, participation entails much of what a paid work position might. Volunteer positions have varying expectations of participation; the level at which this occurs varies according to the role the volunteer plays and the organization. A volunteer who leads a weekly community yoga class will have different expectations than those of the president of the AOTA (a volunteer position!). The demands for those activities involved should match the volunteer's abilities and time available (as was addressed in the precursor to this occupation–volunteer exploration).

Play

"Any spontaneous or organized activity that provides enjoyment, entertainment, amusement, or diversion" (Parham & Fazio, 1997, p. 252).

What defines *play* and how it is different from *leisure* has been a debate evident in the literature for years. Definitions of *play* range from focusing on the activities of children to spontaneous action that provides enjoyment. However, if observing a group of adults playing laser tag, one can assert that no one definition seems appropriate. At what point in human development do we stop playing and start engaging in leisure? While play is the primary occupation of children, it is an occupation that can be engaged in across the lifespan.

Play and its impact on humans has been an area of study for many scientists who have identified some key elements of play that correspond and are agreed upon by most theories and definitions of play. Play activities are engaged upon for intrinsic rewards, such as happiness or excitement, not for external rewards or gains. Play is also focused on the process or the "doing" of the activity versus an end result. Play activities are also those that are freely chosen, not engaged in because of expectations or requirements. The most essential characteristic of play is that it provides enjoyment or pleasure (Parham, 2008). While other occupations may provoke these emotions, play is not possible without enjoyment or pleasure and is the primary motivator toward engagement in play. For example, we may feel enjoyment or pleasure while cooking or working, but it is not the primary motivator towards why we engage in it. For some people, cooking can have many traits of play but is a leisure or IADL activity due to the fact that the focus is on the end result of what is prepared. We will further define the characteristics of leisure later in this chapter.

Play Exploration

"Identifying appropriate play activities, which can include exploration play, practice play, pretend play, games with rules, constructive play, and symbolic play (adapted from Bergen, 1988, pp. 64–65)" (AOTA, 2008, p. 632).

To thoroughly understand the scope and breadth of the complexity of play, one could read hundreds of books and journals on the topic. The *Framework* introduces us to some of the basic concepts of play and the different forms that the occupation of play can take. Play exploration is differentiated as an occupation separate from participation in play, in that play exploration activities are the child's or adult's actions toward investigating and choosing play activities. A child may begin one play activity, and then shift to another based on intrinsic needs or developmental level. When involved in social play (play conducted with others), play exploration requires collaborating with other children or adults to determine the play activities.

The *Framework* presents six different types of play that have been named and defined by different theories. Jean Piaget, a developmental psychologist, fathered foundational theories that emphasized

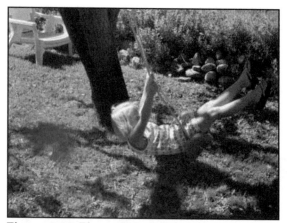

Figure 2-11. Play: symbolic play.

that cognitive development occurred out of play experiences. Over the years, other theorists have utilized Piaget's play theory as a basis for development of other theories which include fundamental aspects of how the play experience contributes to human development. Out of these theories, several categories or types of play have been identified, which change as a child develops and ages (Knox, 2005).

Practice play, which typically occurs from infancy to 2 years of age, includes activities that are conducted for the sake of experiencing the effect. This is often termed *sensorimotor play* as this type of play includes exploring sensations and how the body moves (Parham, 2008). Mary Reilly termed this type of play *exploratory play*, which she believed to encompass more than cognitive development, and is a means by which a child seeks to understand his or her environment and sensory experiences (Parham, 2008). This type of play behavior is strictly intrinsically motivated, as this is how a child comes to understand how to move his or her body to create actions or have an effect on his or her environment. This is also how he or she creates an understanding of sensory characteristics, such as sights, sounds, and motions. Examples of exploratory play include playing with rattles, balls, blocks, mobiles, squeeze toys, and small puzzles.

In symbolic play, the child begins to understand how objects are used and how they can control and manipulate objects to create action or change. Primarily gross motor activities, such as playing with dough, finger painting, puzzles, tumbling, riding a tricycle, or playing on swings (Figure 2-11), the child learns how to move and formulate concepts about the world around them. Simple art activities such as coloring or use of chalk, glue, or stringing beads are just a few examples of the emergence of fine motor activities in play. Interactions with others may also be part of symbolic play, assisting with language development and understanding human

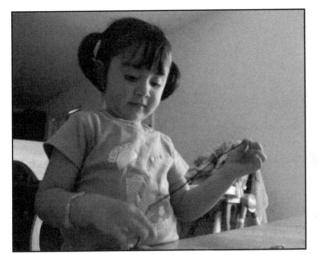

Figure 2-12. Play: constructive play.

relationships. This type of play begins at age 1 and continues to increase up to age 5 (Knox, 2005). Constructive play occurs when the child begins to utilize objects to build and create. Materials used for this type of play range from crayons and paper, to baking cookies or stringing beads (Figure 2-12). This is also termed *creative play* as this is when imagination and creative expression is exhibited. Creative and constructive play typically begins at 4 to 7 years of age (Morrison, Metzger, & Pratt, 1996).

Pretend play begins to occur during the second year and continues to increase up to age 7, at which point it begins to taper off in occurrence (Munier, Myers, & Pierce, 2008). This type of play involves the child imitating or mimicking actions that may or may not occur in the real world. For example, a child may tie a towel around his or her neck creating a cape and imagining and acting as if he or she is a superhero. Playing with dolls and pretending to cook or prepare a tea party are examples of pretend play. Children often imitate sounds that they believe are created during the action that occurs, such as the sound cars or trucks make when racing and then crashing into each other.

Playing games with distinct rules occurs in children 7 to 12 years of age. These games require social interaction and have consequences to actions. These play activities can include structured games such as checkers, card games, or jump rope. Unstructured play activities that have social rules such as cooking or pet care are also considered games with rules. Creating specific objects that require following directions such as creating arts and crafts objects or models also falls under this type of play, as it requires following rules in order to complete the task. Peers, parents, or other adults facilitate the rules and social interaction during these activities (Knox, 2005).

Play Participation

"Participating in play; maintaining a balance of play with other areas of occupation; and obtaining, using, and maintaining, toys, equipment, and supplies appropriately" (AOTA, 2008, p. 632).

Engaging in play is part of human development, facilitating cognitive, perceptual, and physical skill development that is needed to become a mature adult. Without an adequate opportunity to participate in play, a child will not be given the opportunity to develop the skills that emerge from engaging in play. For example, if a child is secluded from other children for the first 6 years of his or her life, he or she will not learn the social skills necessary to socialize with others at that developmental level. Thus, engagement in play is essential to a child's life and must be balanced with other occupations that occupy the day.

Play activities are defined by the child or adult participating in them and the environment and culture that surround them. Thus, the variety of activities that comprise play is wide-ranging and diverse. Play activities require varying levels of physical, mental, and social engagement, utilizing a range of objects, toys, or equipment. For one child, play may include making army men out of sticks, while another uses a computer to play video games. Play participation includes the activities surrounding obtaining and properly utilizing the objects used in play activities. In some play activities, the child will manipulate an object or the environment, such as shaking a rattle or digging in dirt.

The maintenance of toys and other objects used during play is considered part of the play experience. In order to participate in the play activity, the child must not only gain access to materials or objects but also maintain possession of the objects in order to continue playing. For example, if a child is engaged in painting but decides to pour the paint into the toilet, the play activity of painting cannot continue. Understanding how to maintain objects and materials in order to continue play activities emerges after a child has developed the concepts of cause and effect and insight.

Leisure

"A nonobligatory activity that is intrinsically motivated and engaged in during discretionary time, that is time not committed to obligatory occupations such as work, self-care, or sleep" (Parham & Fazio, 1997, p. 250).

How leisure is different from play is a debate that has been portrayed in the literature for decades. There are more similarities between the two than differences.

Activity 2-4

Think about the activities that you do in your spare time, which do not include ADL, IADL, or other obligatory occupations (those activities that you must do). Next to each activity, describe in a few words how participating in this activity makes you feel. This should also reflect why you chose to participate in the activity.

	Activity	**Rewards**
1.		
2.		
3.		
4.		
5.		

Play activities are different from leisure in that play is a vital aspect of child development, while leisure is not related to human development in children or adults (Deitz & Swinth, 2008). However, leisure activities are intrinsically motivating to participate in, meaning there is some emotional reward (which may include enjoyment, entertainment, amusement, or diversion). The most defining aspect of leisure is that it is a nonobligatory activity, which means it is not an activity that addresses other needs in life. Leisure activity is done simply for enjoyment or to meet other intrinsic needs.

Leisure Exploration

"Identifying interests, skills, opportunities, and appropriate leisure activities" (AOTA, 2008, p. 632).

Leisure exploration is the process of finding activities that meet intrinsic needs and are activities that are not obligatory toward other aspects of living (such as self-care, child care, home maintenance, etc.). Identifying activities requires seeking out a match of a person's interests, intrinsic needs, and abilities to leisure opportunities. A person who is seeking out leisure opportunities will learn about possible activities by talking to others, watching the activity, watching information about the activity on the television, or searching the Internet. Exploring activities does not necessarily lead to participation. For example, a person may spend time investigating how to take skydiving lessons but find that the personal expense (and fright) outweighs the personal benefits and choose not to follow through with the idea.

Leisure Participation

"Planning and participating in appropriate leisure activities; maintaining a balance of leisure activities with other areas of occupation; and

obtaining, using, and maintaining equipment and supplies as appropriate" (AOTA, 2008, p. 632).

As discussed earlier, leisure is defined as those activities that comprise nonobligatory time and are intrinsically rewarding. How we choose to spend our spare time (discretionary time) is unique to each individual and changes over the lifespan. Think about the activities you did when you were in high school that you considered fun outside of the educational setting (not related to school). You may still engage in some of these activities, while you may have discarded others for new ones as you matured. Participating in leisure activities is an important part of living a balanced life throughout the lifespan, regardless of physical or mental abilities or age. Allowing for an adequate balance of time to engage in leisure activities may be deprived due to busy schedules, limited income, or restrictive environment (such as with those in prisons or the homeless).

Leisure activities range from active to quiet or sedentary activities. Active activities are those that require active movement within the environment or outdoors. Hiking, shopping, gardening, bike riding, and swimming are just a few examples of active leisure activities. Quiet or sedentary activities are those that require little motor movement and may be done sitting or with small amounts of walking. Examples of sedentary leisure activities are reading, surfing the Internet, watching television, or knitting. Each type provides its own intrinsic rewards, such as happiness, excitement, pride, or self-efficacy. Complete Activity 2-4 to get an idea of what motivates you toward participation in leisure activities.

Participating in leisure activities also requires adequate preparation by preparing the self, environment, and objects used. For example, before going for a hike, one must first determine where the hike will take place and how to get there. The

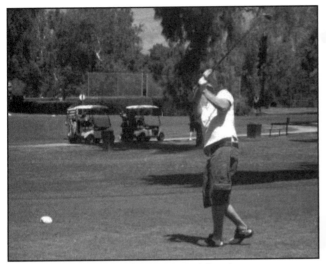

Figure 2-13. Leisure: leisure participation

objects needed must be gathered, such as a map, water, snacks, and walking stick (if needed). The person hiking will prepare him- or herself for the hike by donning the appropriate clothing and shoes. Preparing the body for the hike may also include applying insect repellent or sunscreen. All of these preparatory activities are part of leisure, as they are not linked to other obligatory activities. Maintaining the equipment and objects used during the leisure activity is also part of participation, as it again is not linked to other obligatory occupations and allows for future leisure participation. In other words, assuring that equipment and supplies are kept in usable condition allows the person to use the equipment again in the future. For example, when Vern goes golfing, he assures that when he is done he cleans each of the golf clubs and puts them back into their proper place. He cleans the spikes in his golf shoes and puts all of the tees away. This way, when he wants to go golfing again, he has all of the equipment he needs and it will be in working order (Figure 2-13).

Social Participation

"Activities associated with organized patterns of behavior that are characteristic and expected of an individual or an individual or an individual interacting with others within a given social system (adapted from Mosey, 1996, p. 340)" (AOTA, 2008, p. 633).

Community

"Activities that result in successful interaction at the community level (i.e., neighborhood, organizations, work, school)" (AOTA, 2008, p. 633).

Social interactions at a community level are those that connect two or more individuals together as a group. Communities of people occur within many arenas outside of the home, such as at school, at work, within the neighborhood, or possibly at church or other organizations. Social participation includes not only verbally communicating but engaging in activities together. The interactions that occur and are required to be part of vary according to the social rules of the group. Topics of conversation and how a person acts around others are parts of the social rules that are embedded in the activities surrounding social participation. Socially interacting with others may include physical interactions with each other, such as a hug when meeting or sharing equipment or objects. Interaction can also occur when not face to face with others. Online communities and e-mail are part of community-based social participation, in which there is a very different set of expectations than when interacting in person. Interacting with a person or a group within an online community may include rules such as not using obscene language or pictures, not using all capital letters when writing a sentence, and responding to others in a respectful manner.

Social participation on a community level is different from that at the family or peer level. For example, Jenny participates socially with her coworkers on a level that is different from that with her friends. During breaks and lunches, she and her coworkers joke about their clients and struggles from the day, while lightly touching on personal topics. Jenny uses terms that her coworkers are familiar with as they all work in the public relations business. Jenny also will attend after-work events to further the bond with her coworkers, such as attending a beach bonfire party. While Jenny may refer to some of the people she interacts with as "friends," they are all coworkers and the social activities, which are work related, are at a community level.

Family

"[Activities that result in] successful interaction in specific required and/or desired familial roles" (Mosey, 1996, p. 340).

Activities involving family interactions are often embedded in culture and tradition (Figure 2-14). Each family will have its own expectations for communication and interaction, based on each individual's role within the family. A son may interact with a father differently than with his mother, based on the expectations within his family. Social interaction between family members can occur one-on-one or as a group and does not necessarily occur in person.

Just as with social participation within a community, social participation within families can occur via the Internet or phone. Social interactions with family members often surround daily activities such as meal preparation, child rearing, and self-feeding. If living with family members, social participation may occur throughout all activities that include the home environment. A child who has many siblings will need to engage socially with his or her brothers and sisters continuously as he or she engages in self-care, play, and possibly educational occupations. They must communicate their needs, share objects and space, and physically interact with their siblings throughout many of these activities.

Jun is 34 and engages in a variety of social activities, each dependent on her familial role. As a daughter, she calls on her mom every morning, to see how she is feeling and if she needs her to pick up anything from the store. She then wakes up her 4-year-old daughter, singing to her. She wakes up her 2-year-old son by giving him big hugs and tickling him. When she sees her father, she greets him with a hug and a kiss and her interactions with him are filled with respect, turning to him for advice and wisdom. The conversations she has with each of her family members is unique and has its own set of physical interactions. The example of Jun is only a glimpse of how one family interacts; how each family interacts and socially engages in activities together is developed over time and is different for each family unit.

Peer, Friend

"Activities at different levels of intimacy, including engaging in desired sexual activity" (AOTA, 2008, p. 633).

Engaging socially with our friends, peers, lovers, and acquaintances occurs in many avenues of our lives, in many different ways. We might engage in "small talk" about the weather to an acquaintance or someone we just met at a party, while we might cry on the shoulder of a good friend and tell of our deepest woes. Engaging with others not only occurs in the community, workplace, and within family groups but in solitary relationships with those whom we see as peers. Activities involving social participation with friends or peers often occur within other occupations such as talking with a friend while shopping together or sharing a joke while riding on a ski lift. Engagement in social activities is reflected in interactions between two people, how their bodies move in relation to each other, and sharing the experience of engaging in an occupation together. The occupations can be very intimate, such as sexual activity, or purely platonic, such as sharing a meal together. The type

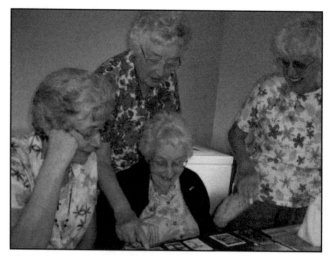

Figure 2-14. Social participation: family.

of relationship held between two people determines the intensity and level of social participation. It is the engagement in social activities that establishes, maintains, or destroys the relationship. Friendships are developed by engaging in conversation and shared experiences. The friendship is maintained by actions made toward each person, with continued action with both people involved. For example, Mercedes and Alison met at a mutual friend's party. They began talking to each other about their children and found that they had much in common. At the end of the night, they exchanged e-mail addresses. Shortly after, they met up for coffee. Now, they call or e-mail each other once a week and occasionally go for a walk or meet up for breakfast. The actions Alison made to connect with Mercedes, and those made by Mercedes to Alison, were all social participation activities.

Conclusion

Determining what to analyze and paring it down to a workable activity is the first step to activity analysis (Activity 2-5). This requires having an understanding of what defines success by the client or as the activity is typically done if conducting a standard activity analysis. The *Framework* has helped clinicians in defining occupations and the scope of our practice by creating major categories of occupations and defining what activities are part of each of those categories through the areas of occupation section of the *Framework*. This can be used in activity analysis to help the clinician define in what area of occupation the activity is classified, as well as helping to gain an understanding of all of the tasks that are part of the activity.

Activity 2-5

Indicate which area(s) of occupation each activity or task would be categorized as:

	ADL	IADL	Education	Work	Play	Leisure	Social participation
Surf the Web							
Organize your CD collection							
Ride a bike							
Fold laundry							
Pour a cup of coffee							
Sing in the shower							
Put on ski boots							
Throw a party							
Put gas in the car							
Get newspaper from yard							
Cut coupons							
Take a bubble bath							
Smoke a cigarette							
Go to church							
Water plants							
Pick lint out of belly button							

The purpose of this exercise was to get you thinking about the different areas of occupation and being able to identify which categories different activities might fall under. There is also another hidden objective behind this activity. Compare your answers to some of your classmates' answers. Are they different? Why? This exercise shows how the meaning behind occupations can be different for each individual. For example, I consider organizing a CD collection as an IADL, as home establishment and management (it is not a fun task for me). However, if you asked my husband, he would consider this leisure as well. He enjoys doing this and painstakingly alphabetizes each CD with glee. It is a requirement of home establishment and management but also has leisure aspects of it for him. If I asked you to categorize the activity of painting a picture, would you consider that leisure? As an OT student, it could be leisure or part of a class and thus classified under "formal education participation." But let's say you have a client who is a professional artist. Painting is now considered work. Thus, the areas of occupation are best utilized when conducting occupation-based activity analyses (within the contexts of an individual).

QUESTIONS

1. What is the purpose of the areas of occupation section of the *Framework*?

2. How is feeding different from eating?

3. What is the difference between a prosthetic and an orthotic? How are these part of activities of daily living?

4. What are ways in which community mobility is conducted?

5. What are at least three activities that would be considered retirement preparation?

6. What activities would be considered "play" if an adult was the participant?

7. List three social participation activities.

ACTIVITY

1. What is the range of occupations in which humans engage? Using a variety of magazines, cut out pictures of people engaging in occupations. As a class, create eight poster boards, one for each area of occupation. The class can divide up into groups, each addressing an area of occupation. Once completed, share each board—the visual representation of the broad spectrum of activities that are included in each area. Collectively, all of these boards represent the domain of OT and can be displayed for others to see.

REFERENCES

American Occupational Therapy Association. (2008). Occupational therapy practice framework: Domain and process (2nd ed.). *American Journal of Occupational Therapy, 62,* 625–683.

Billock, C. (2009). Spirituality, occupation, and occupational therapy. In E. Crepeau, E. Cohn, B. Boyt Schell, (Eds.). *Willard and Spackman's occupational therapy,* (11th ed., pp. 90–96). Philadelphia, PA: Lippincott Williams & Wilkins.

Christiansen, C., & Hammecker, C. (2001). Self care. In B.R. Bonder & M.B. Wagner (Eds.), *Functional performance in older adults* (pp. 155–715). Philadelphia: F.A. Davis

Cook, A., & Hussey, S. (2002). *Assistive technologies: Principles and practice* (2nd ed.). St. Louis, MO: Mosby, Inc.

Dave, D., Rashad, I., & Spasojevic, J. (2008). The effects of retirement on physical and mental health outcomes. *Southern Economic Journal, 75*(2), 497–524.

Deitz, J., & Swinth, Y. (2008). Accessing play through assistive technology. In L.D. Parham & L. Fazio (Eds.), *Play in occupational therapy for children* (2nd ed., pp. 395–412). St. Louis, MO: Mosby Elsevier.

Deshaies, L. (2008). Upper extremity orthoses. In M. Radomski & C. Trombly Latham (Eds.), *Occupational therapy for physical dysfunction* (6th ed., pp. 421–464). Baltimore, MD: Lippincott Williams & Wilkins.

Hagedorn, R. (1995). *Occupational therapy, perspectives and processes.* Edinburgh, UK: Churchill Livingstone.

Hagedorn, R. (1997). *Foundations for practice in occupational therapy.* Edinburgh, UK: Churchill Livingstone.

Hinojosa, J., Kramer, P., & Pratt, P. (1996). Foundations of practice: Developmental principles, theories, and frames of reference. In J. Case-Smith, A. Allen, & P. Pratt (Eds.), *Occupational therapy for children* (3rd ed., pp. 25–45). St. Louis, MO: Mosby.

Knox, S. (2005). Play. In J. Case-Smith (Ed.), *Occupational therapy for children* (5th ed., pp. 571–586). St. Louis, MO: Mosby Elsevier.

McKnight-Eily, L., Presley-Cantrell, L., Strine, T., Chapman, D., Perry, G. & Croft, J. (2008). Perceived insufficient rest or sleep—Four states. *Morbidity and Mortality Weekly, 57*(8), 200–203.

McMinn, A. (2009). Active retirement for healthier aging. *Perspectives in Public Health, 129*(4), 158–160.

Moriera-Almeida, A., & Koenig, H. G. (2006). Retaining the meaning of the words religiousness and spirituality: A commentary on the WHOQOL SRPB group's "A cross-cultural study of spirituality, religion, and personal beliefs as components of quality of life." *Social Science and Medicine, 62*(6), 843–844.

Morrison, C., Metzger, P. & Pratt, P. (1996). Play. In J. Case-Smith, A. Allen, & P. Pratt (Eds.), *Occupational therapy for children* (3rd ed., pp. 504–524). St. Louis, MO: Mosby.

Mosby's dictionary of medicine, nursing & health professions. (2006). St. Louis, MO: Mosby Elsevier.

Mosey, A. (1996). *Applied scientific inquiry in the health professions: An epistemological orientation* (2nd ed.). Bethesda, MD: American Occupational Therapy Association.

Moyers P., & Dale, L. (2007). *The guide to occupational therapy practice* (2nd ed.). Bethesda, MD: AOTA Press.

Munier, V., Myers, C., & Pierce, D. (2008). Power of object play for infants and toddlers. In L.D. Parham & L. Fazio (Eds.), *Play in occupational therapy for children,* (2nd ed., pp. 219–249). St. Louis, MO: Mosby Elsevier.

Nurit, W., & Michel, A. (2003). Rest: A qualitative exploration of the phenomenon. *Occupational Therapy International, 10,* 227–238.

Parham, L. D. (2008). Play and occupational therapy. In L. D. Parham & L. Fazio (Eds.), *Play in occupational therapy for children* (2nd ed., pp. 3–39). St. Louis, MO: Mosby Elsevier.

Parham, L., & Fazio, L. (Eds.). (1997). *Play in occupational therapy for children.* St. Louis, MO: Mosby.

Rogers, J., & Holm, M. (1994). Assessment of self-care. In B. R. Bonder & M.B. Wagner (Eds.), *Functional performance in older adults* (pp. 181–202). Philadelphia, PA: F. A. Davis.

West, L. (2009). Sleep: An emerging practice area? *OT Practice, 14*(8), 9-10.

World Health Organization. (2001). *International classification of functioning, disability, and health.* Geneva, Switzerland: Author.

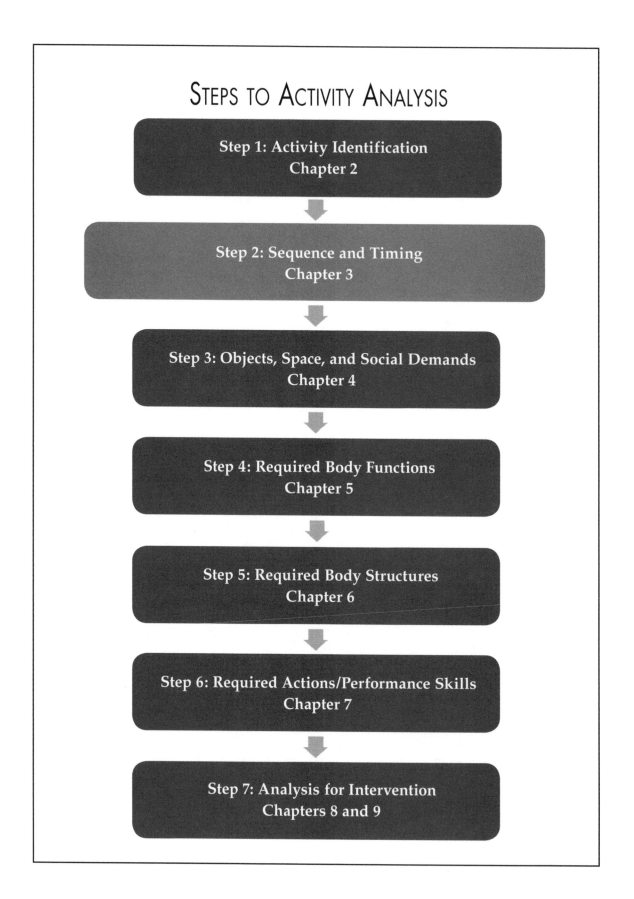

STEPS TO ACTIVITY ANALYSIS

Step 1: Activity Identification
Chapter 2

Step 2: Sequence and Timing
Chapter 3

Step 3: Objects, Space, and Social Demands
Chapter 4

Step 4: Required Body Functions
Chapter 5

Step 5: Required Body Structures
Chapter 6

Step 6: Required Actions/Performance Skills
Chapter 7

Step 7: Analysis for Intervention
Chapters 8 and 9

3

SEQUENCE AND TIMING

OBJECTIVES

1. Identify methods in which to determine the sequence and timing of steps to an activity.

2. Determine the positive and negative aspects of each method for determining steps to an activity.

3. List the elements to be included when using procedural task analysis to list the steps of an activity.

4. Understand how co-occupations exist within occupations of clients.

5. Define how occupations can be nested within other occupations.

In order to understand an activity, and the demands that activity would place on a person performing that activity, one must first clearly identify what the activity being analyzed is and then break that activity down into its component steps. Each step holds information that may be the key to successful performance. For example, if analyzing the activity of washing hands, a key step is using the soap. This requires reaching for the soap, grasping it (assuming it is a bar of soap), bringing it to the other hand, and moving the bar over both hands. Looking at each of these steps adds a new action and challenge for the person performing the task. Activity analysis is used during the evaluation, intervention, and outcome measurement and thus is essential to practice. Being able to identify the steps and timing for an activity is what leads to successful analysis.

ESSENTIAL STEPS TOWARD SUCCESS

Determining the essential steps to success will help you with this part of the activity analysis process. While each person may complete an activity differently than the next person, it is important to understand which steps or timing elements are essential for successful performance of an activity. What defines *success*? For most activities, there are clear ways to determine success, which often include being able to move on to each step. An example of this is turning on the water as an essential step to taking a shower. Without this step, and in the correct order, the step following this would not allow a person to be able to shower. While in this example the essential step is easy to see, in many cases the essential steps may seem subjective or rely on what the client sees as successful completion. In the example of showering, a client may not see the use of washing the hair with shampoo during the shower as an essential step. This is where it is important to define the activity clearly. Washing the hair can be seen as a separate activity that is "nested" within the activity of showering (we will talk about nesting later in this chapter). Perhaps your client does not wash his or her own hair but has it shampooed and styled at a salon. So, what defines showering? For this activity, the *Occupational Therapy Practice Framework, 2nd Edition* (*Framework*) nicely defines for us what this entails—obtaining and using supplies, soaping, rinsing, and drying body parts (American Occupational Therapy Association [AOTA], 2008). However, what if we are analyzing an activity that is not defined in the *Framework*? Let's

Thomas, H. *Occupation-Based Activity Analysis* (pp. 39-47).
© 2012 SLACK Incorporated

take a look at the activity of cleaning a cat's litter box. We begin by clearly stating the activity in a way that delineates what is expected from the activity: all feline waste is removed from the litter box, leaving only clean litter. You might need to define activities in this manner for your clients, so that it is clear as to what is expected. "Please clean and dry your entire body in the shower," is an example.

METHODS FOR DETERMINING KEY STEPS

Once you have clearly defined the activity, you must now begin to list the key steps. Experience may allow us to mentally recall the steps of an activity that is familiar to us, but it is impossible to know the details of every occupation known to humankind. For example, you may have a client who is hoping to return to his job as a pharmacist. Understanding the activities required of this profession, as well as the steps to each of the activities, can be found in several ways. There are pros and cons to each method for determining the steps required of an activity; however, the method we choose may have much to do with pragmatic factors such as cost and time.

Mentally Process the Steps

With simple, everyday tasks, the easiest way to determine the steps is to mentally visualize each step. For example, if asked what the component steps are to washing your hands, you would probably be able to come up with the essential steps. However, with more complex activities, this may not be feasible. By simply relying on your own memory and understanding of an activity, many steps may be left out. The benefits of this method are that it takes very little time or expense. It is a technique that clinicians use continuously throughout their day, planning intervention sessions, conducting evaluations, and discharge planning with clients. Through experience, practice, and exposure to common occupations, the ability to mentally visualize steps evolves and the ease in which this occurs improves.

Engage in the Activity Yourself

While not always possible, engaging in the activity yourself gives you a perspective not possible with other methods. While the experience of an activity is different for each person, participating in an activity allow you to "feel" what it is like to participate in the activity and pick up on steps and elements that may not be detected through mental visualization or by watching others. There may be timing elements that are difficult to determine, such as the exact moment

something should happen or the next step should occur. For example, if you were to write down the sequence and timing of flying a kite, you would probably be able to come up with the basic sequence (if you had ever engaged in this activity). But if I gave you a kite and asked you to set it into flight, you would find there are many elements of timing that are not evident when just watching someone else do it or mentally visualizing it. To get the kite up into the air, you must use the air flow, which is felt through the kite string. By pulling on the kite string at the right time, the kite will glide up on air currents. Understanding this complex sequence and timing and the actions required is not easily "seen" but is felt. This is true of many occupations. It is often difficult to break down an occupation into a sequence of actions when the actions are not observable, or each step is reliant on external occurrences, or the outcome of a previous step.

Participating in an occupation or activity allows the clinician to gather a broader understanding of an activity, allowing for a more accurate analysis. It allows us to creatively find activities that meet our client's needs. If working with a client who has weak supinators, how might you find an activity that would require him to supinate his hand? As you sit reading this, are you supinating your hand, perhaps mimicking movements of activities? If you were to try to find an activity that requires this motion, you could begin trials of different things yourself. Does playing cards, brushing teeth, folding paper, or using a phone challenge the supinators? (Ok, try these.)

There are as many limitations to this method as there are benefits. Time is often the greatest limitation. Unfortunately, we do not always have the time to experience all of the occupations that our clients do (our employers are also hesitant to pay us to do so). Especially in the case of occupations that span great lengths of time, participating in them ourselves is not always possible. The contexts in which the occupations occur also limit our participation. For example, let's say we are analyzing the activity of ice climbing (Figure 3-1). The physical environment in which this occurs requires that we be in a climate that is cold (very cold) and have a surface covered in ice in which to climb. Ice climbing is typically done in pairs or with groups, in which there are social expectations of participation. There is also special equipment needed, such as spikes to clamp onto boots, a helmet, ropes, and other protective gear. There is also a certain amount of skill and body functions that are required to safely climb ice and survive. The demands of this activity, and many activities that our clients participate in, limit our choice of method in which we can analyze the activity. Participating in

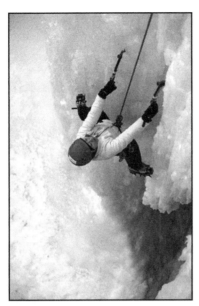

Figure 3-1. Ice climbing Canadian Rockies. (Photo by B. Jardine. Reprinted with permission of Yamnuska Mountain Adventures.)

activity ourselves is not only limited by time and cost but by safety, knowledge of the clinician, physical environment, and access to the tools and equipment.

Talk to Your Client

The person most intimately involved in an occupation is going to be your client. Asking your client to explain an activity step by step may give you an overall idea of how a task is done and the objects and equipment needed. The client may be able to give you information regarding aspects of the activity that cannot be seen by an observer. However, you must keep in mind that your client may leave out essential details, assuming that you already know about certain aspects of the activity or because he or she is unsure of how much detail to give you. Some clients may be unable to verbally give you the information needed, due to cognitive or speech impairments. However, this is often the easiest and quickest way to gather information. When time and travel are delimiters, asking the client is often the most feasible option. If asking the client to give you information regarding an activity, it is important that you ask probing questions to gather all of the pertinent details. Use the activity demands section of the *Framework* to guide you. For example, ask about the objects and properties such as the size, shape, and weight of the objects used. If your client states that he or she uses a hammer, ask what type, how big, how heavy, and what shape the handle is. If the client states that he or she works in a garage,

ask for a description of that space in regards to not only the size but the lighting, temperature, noise, and ventilation.

Talk to Someone Who Performs This Activity

When talking to the client is not feasible or does not give you enough information, talking to another person who performs that activity can often prove to give valuable information. In the example of the client who is a pharmacist, gathering information from the client's coworkers or employer would be a valid strategy for finding out what the activity demands are in his job responsibilities. If utilizing this strategy, it is best to be prepared with a list of questions for the person you are talking to. Be ready to ask very pointed questions to allow you to gather all of the needed information at one time. Just as was the case with talking to your client, you may find that the person you talk to may not give much detail or leave key elements out of their description because they assume you already know certain elements. Preface your conversation with a brief explanation of what you are looking for and the depth of your current understanding of the activities you will be discussing. Be respectful of the person's time and be prepared to be flexible to what time they are able to give you. This is one of the limitations of this method—coordinating time between the clinician and the experienced person. It may be difficult to find someone willing to talk with you, especially in situations where the occupation or activity is uncommon (such as making prosthetic eyes), participants of the occupation are very busy (the mother of quadruplets) or the information is seen as private information (the activities of a monk from a certain sect). You may find cultural or language barriers to gathering the information. Those you attempt to talk to may not understand why you are asking or may be hesitant to share information with you. For example, several years ago, I had the privilege of working with a gentleman who had had a stroke and was a practicing monk. The garment he wore everyday was an elaborate robe that wrapped around the body in different directions. One of the primary goals in occupational therapy (OT) was to learn how to put on this robe by himself, despite the fact that he only had the use of one hand. Due to his physical and speech limitations from the stroke, he was unable to show me how the material from the gown was to be wrapped. When a group of fellow monks from his monastery came to visit him in the hospital, I asked about the robe-wrapping process. The group of men looked offended, and many of them looked away. I found that they were not allowed to talk to women and that the process of donning the robe is a sacred and private process that is not shared with others. Respectful of their beliefs, I had a male therapist explain to them the reason for my asking, and one of the monks agreed to work with the patient on this task.

Watch Someone Perform the Activity

Watching your client or another person perform an activity can give you great information on the physical actions required as well as the timing and sequence of steps. Through careful observation, the clinician can gather information regarding strength, range of movements, coordination, and duration of movements required. The clinician can also begin to get a sense of the mental, sensory, and speech functions required. This method works well in situations where the experience of the clinician is a limiting factor or the context of the activity does not lend itself to be analyzed in other ways. While observing your client participating in the activity may give you some information, you may need to observe another person participating in the activity if your client is not able to perform the activity completely or you need further information than your client can provide for you. If you find another person performing the activity (in a similar context as your client), ask the person if you can observe them. Explain the purpose for your observation and obtain permission to take notes. You may also choose to videotape the activity. This allows you to rewind and slowly analyze aspects of the activity at your own pace. Keep in mind that you may need to receive written permission from those you are videotaping unless in a public forum. You may be able to find video information on the activity without having to record it yourself. In the example of the activity of ice climbing, the clinician can observe others in two ways—in person or by video. Ice climbing videos abound on the Internet and are available on DVD or video. This is a more cost- and time-efficient method for analyzing the activity. However, the timing, sequencing, and actions used by another person may not always be the same used by your client, and this should always be considered when conducting an occupation-based activity analysis.

PROCEDURAL TASK ANALYSIS: DETERMINING SEQUENCE AND TIMING

Yuen and D'Amico (1998) described a technique called *procedural task analysis* which is used by OT practitioners to help determine the sequence of steps for an activity. Their suggestions for this process provide excellent guidelines for determining the sequence and timing of an activity. While the *Framework* does not detail the process to determine the sequence and timing (Table 3 of the *Framework*), adopting a method that lends itself to a more accurate description of the essential steps leads to a precise analysis of the activity demands and greater ability to explain to or teach a client or caregiver. Thus, the suggestions of Yuen and D'Amico will be used as a guide for writing out the sequence and timing for an activity analysis.

1. Determine what activity you will be analyzing. Be sure to break down larger occupations into smaller activities or tasks, so that the analysis will be much more feasible and understandable. For example, instead of analyzing the activity of skiing, you may choose to analyze one component, such as purchasing a lift ticket or getting on a ski lift.

2. Preparatory and clean up tasks should only be included in the steps if absolutely necessary. Otherwise, these can be separate activities. For example, you may not want to list all of the step required for getting prepared to play a board game; however, you might want to list the preparatory steps for a computer task (i.e., turn on the computer).

3. When writing out a step, be sure to begin the statement with an action verb. This verb describes what the person participating in the activity must do. These actions should be observable. Examples of action verbs are *grab, open, write, step.*

4. The next part of the statement should include what the objects or environmental aspects are being acted upon. In the statement: "squeeze the bottle," *squeeze* is the action verb and *bottle* is the object.

5. One of the most important aspects of the statement is *how* the action should be completed. This can be a simple word such as *slowly* or more descriptive such as "in the shape of a figure-eight." These descriptors can be placed at the beginning of the statement, at the end, or both. For example, "*Carefully* place the pieces of bread together with the *peanut butter and jelly sides going together.*" *Carefully* tells the reader that you cannot slam the two pieces of bread together, and the last half of the statement tells how the pieces should be aligned.

6. Include time elements if the timing of certain steps, or the length of an action, is essential to the task. For example, if making cookies,

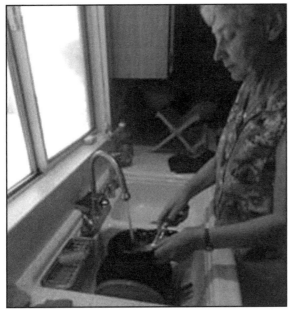

Figure 3-2. Dishes.

you would specify when to take the cookies out of the oven. The directions would state, "Remove the cookies from oven using an oven mitt after 20 minutes." Often the directions are not related to time but other indicators, such as repetitions. For example: "Stir pudding mix 25 times." or "Remove from refrigerator when pudding is a semi-solid and no longer liquid."

Each step should include:

- *Action verb*
- *How the action takes place*
- *Objects used or interacted with*
- *Time elements (if needed)*
- *Amounts used (if needed)*

---

7. List the steps in the correct sequence, as they normally occur. If a step or a sequence of steps reoccurs, state which steps to repeat and for how long. For example: "Repeat steps 3 to 6 until all hair is removed."

8. Keep the steps simple and concise. Keep out unneeded details and avoid including multiple instructions in one step. A sign that you may be including too much information into one step is if there is the word *and* linking two action verbs in your directions. This does not always mean that you are giving two or more steps in

one but is a sign that the direction may be too complex. For example: " Rinse the dishes and then put them in the dishwasher." This is actually two different steps. The first half "rinse the dishes" is the first step that needs further clarification as to how each dish is to be rinsed (and where). The next step would include putting the dish in the dishwasher. An example of where it would be acceptable to combine two actions would be: "Pick up the spatula and place it in the sink." This includes the word *and* and two actions: pick up and place. However, the actions link together into one simple step (Figure 3-2).

9. Be specific as to the amount of a certain material that is needed or used during a step. For example, when describing washing hair, you might state "Pour a quarter-sized amount of shampoo into the opposite hand." Use descriptors if exact amounts such as cups, inches, or numbers are not called for. "Enough to cover the page," "a pinch," "a handful," and "enough to fill the pot" are examples of describing the amount needed for a particular step. While the amount used for a step may seem intrinsically understood to you, for others it may be a novel concept. Jeremy was a young man who suffered a brain injury while skateboarding when he was 17. One of the things he and I worked on was picking out his clothing for the day. I had to be very succinct and specific in the directions that I gave him, as he would often pull out four pairs of underwear, three shirts, and no pants. Until this becomes the new fashion statement of the day, I needed to be more specific about having him choose one of each type of clothing.

10. Some tasks are not as simple as following numbered steps that follow a logical sequence. There are times when the outcome of an action or an environmental situation has implications on the next action taken. This creates conditional statements (or "if-then" statements). If the task you are analyzing has many of these situations occur, or if the participant must make decisions that influence which step is next, you may choose to graph out the steps in an algorithm. An algorithm is a visual diagram of the steps of a task based on information collected during the activity, and then specific options are given for the next step based on that information. Algorithms are used in professions such as mathematics and engineering to help with decision making and to standardize procedures. Health care has

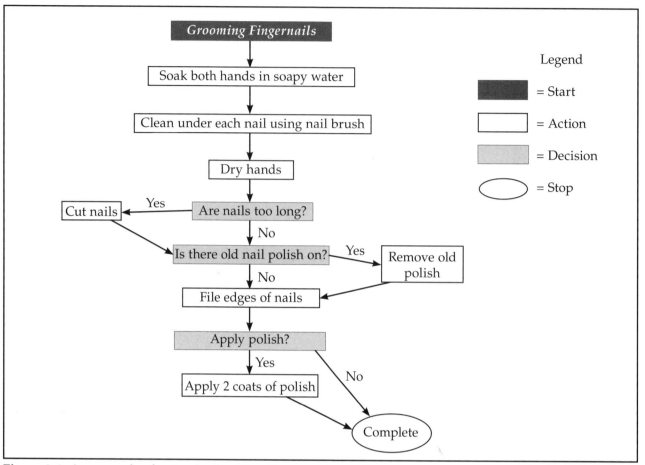

Figure 3-3. An example of a simple algorithm for grooming nails.

used algorithms to design protocols and clinical pathways (Miller, Ryan, & York, 2005). For complex situations, an algorithm can become very large and detailed, especially when there are multiple possible outcomes for each step. The idea behind an algorithm diagram is not to list the details of each step but to help clarify the sequence of steps based on conditional aspects. See Figure 3-3 for an example of a simple algorithm for manicuring nails.

11. Do not indicate to use the right or left hand, unless absolutely necessary. This is also true for which lower extremity to be used for a particular step.

12. Do not list the physical or mental requirement of the task. This part of the analysis comes later and is not included as part of the steps. Write out the steps as if you were going to use the list to instruct a client to do the task. You would not tell a client to "Use vestibular functions to maintain upright position." A good way to check your directions is to read them aloud to

someone, having them act upon each step. If it does not make sense, or the person is not able to act upon your direction, take another look at what you have included in the wording of the directions.

13. Include precautions and warnings for certain steps in parentheses. For example, a statement such as, "Do not touch the metal part of the iron to any body part" could be included in the directions for ironing. Some precautions can be included in part of a step, such as, "Wait 5 minutes or until the polish is dry before using hands to touch objects."

14. Do not include proper nouns or specifics in regards to the objects and properties unless absolutely necessary. For example, you would not state, "Remove nail polish using Smith's heavy-duty polish remover and a cotton ball." In some instances, it is very important to include the name brand or type of material being used, such as in recipes. A recipe for sugar-free cookies may call for the use of a specific sugar

substitute instead of sugar. If a different sugar substitute were used, the amount used might be different, and the end result may not be as successful.

15. While most activities can be completed in many different ways, Lin and Browder (1990) stated that when considering the steps of a task, clinicians must construct the steps in a logical order that considers "sociocultural norms," logical positioning of objects, safety, hygiene, and cost-effectiveness. This means that while you may be able to think of a variety of ways an activity could be done, stick to what is considered the social norm. This would only be done if conducting an activity analysis generically, not an occupation-based activity analysis. When conducting an activity analysis (not an occupation-based activity analysis), be careful to not create special

circumstances or "could be" situations. When listing the steps of an activity, think of how the activity is typically done. As we progress through this book and into Section II, you will see that completing an occupation-based activity analysis will allow you to include the complexities of different situations and ways of completing a task. For now, we are looking at activities in their simpler form as they are generally done by the majority of those who participate in the activity. For example, if asked to list the steps required of making scrambled eggs, you could describe an alternative method of making them in the microwave. However, this is not the typical method used and thus the traditional use of a pan and stove should guide the analysis.

Complete Activity 3-1 to put these to put these principles into practice.

The following is an example of how to write out the sequence and timing for making scrambled eggs (Figure 3-4):

1. Pick up the pan by grasping the handle of the pan with one hand and picking it up.
2. Grasp the can of non-stick spray with the other hand.
3. Hold the nozzle of the can over 6 inches above the pan.
4. Press the nozzle down and spray the entire surface of the pan quickly.
5. Set down the can of spray gently on the countertop.
6. Place the pan on top of the burner.
7. Turn on burner of stove by turning the burner knob to the right slowly until a clicking is heard.
8. Turn the knob to the left slowly until flame is at a medium level.
9. Grasp one egg with one hand.
10. Tap the egg against the edge of the counter until a crack is formed.
11. Bring the egg above the bowl quickly.
12. Using both hands, place thumbs into crack and pull shell apart gently, allowing egg to fall into bowl.
13. Place egg shell into trashcan.
14. Repeat steps 9 to 13 for the second egg
15. Hold the edge of the bowl with the left hand gently.
16. Pick up the fork along the flat edge using right hand.
17. Place fork into bowl and move fork in circular motion quickly.
18. Set fork down onto counter.
19. Pour eggs into pan carefully.

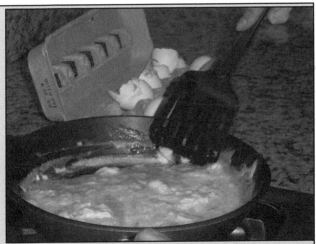

Figure 3-4. Making scrambled eggs.

20. Grasp handle of pan with left hand and pick up spatula with right hand. (Yes, I combined these two steps.)
21. Holding onto handle of pan, stir the eggs slowly with the tip of the spatula.
22. Continue to stir until eggs are fluffy and no longer watery.
23. Turn knob of stove to the off position until the flame goes out.
24. Pick up pan by grasping handle of pan and lifting up carefully.
25. Pick up the spatula along the handle.
26. Tilt pan over the plate and scrape eggs out of pan using the spatula.
27. Set down the pan on the burner.
28. Set down the spatula onto the countertop.

Activity 3-1

1. List out the steps required of washing your hands. Use the following checklist for each step:

    Action verb

    How the action takes place

    Objects used or interacted with

    Time elements (if needed)

    Amounts used (if needed)

    Precautions/warnings

    No right/lefts

    No *ands* linking two action verbs

2. Now ask a classmate or friend to follow your directions as you read them step by step. They are not allowed to assume anything, and must follow your directions exactly as written.

3. Write down which steps are missing or any missing elements. Are there hidden elements that you did not think of?

CO-OCCUPATIONS

Many occupations and activities are not done in solitary and are engaged in with others. Occupations that involve more than one person are called *co-occupations* (Zemke & Clark, 1996). This includes occupations in which social interaction is required or that rely on another person's actions. Caring for a child or a pet is an example of a co-occupation. For example, when David engages in leisure time with his children, the activities in which they engage are reliant on what his children choose. After coming home from a long day at work, David may choose to relax and play with his children, which includes the occupation his children are engaged in—coloring (Figure 3-5).

A similar concept to consider is the idea of nested occupations, in which several occupations are conducted at the same time and co-occur. Co-occupations can be multiple occupations that occur together, such as listening to music and surfing the Internet. Analysis of these types of activities is complex and requires a high level of conditional reasoning that relies on inclusion of the actions of the others participating in the activity. For this reason, listing the sequence and timing of co-occupations is a difficult task. We must recognize that an everyday activity cannot always be reduced to a list of steps. Nevertheless, basic activity analysis gives us the fundamental skills needed to understand the interaction between activity demands and participation in occupations.

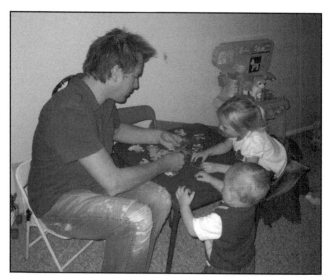

Figure 3-5. Co-occupation.

CONCLUSION

The process of breaking down an activity into its component parts is essential to understanding the complexity of an activity. It includes identifying those aspects of the activity you can see, such as actions, as well as those you do not, such as waiting for a specific amount of time. It is important to identify those steps that are essential to successful participation and completion of the activity and the importance of the order in which they occur. There are many different methods by which to gather this information; some methods offer greater depth but require more time, while those that require less time and effort tend to lack accuracy. Each step of the activity should include an action, description of how the action takes place, objects used or interacted with, and time elements (if needed). Describing the steps needed becomes more complex when others are involved, such as in co-occupations, where actions of one person rely on the actions of another.

QUESTIONS

1. Why is it important to find out the steps required of an activity?

2. Fold a piece of paper in half lengthwise. On one half write down all of the steps required of brushing teeth at the sink. Take those directions and read them to another person, having him or her follow each command exactly. Were there any steps missing? Now on the other half of the paper have the person go step by step through brushing his or her teeth and write down the steps as you observe them. How are the steps you wrote down this time different than when you did it the first time?

3. List at least five things essential to determining the correct sequence and timing.

4. What are examples of co-occupations?

ACTIVITY

1. Analyze the activity of shampooing your hair in the shower. Write out each step in the correct format, numbering each step. Analyze it as it is typically done, all supplies in the shower (shampoo only, no conditioner).

2. You are working with a client who wants to return to the occupation of racing pine box derby cars. Using your favorite Internet browser, find videos that will give you information on how this is done (also called pine wood derby cars). Write out the steps as described in this chapter.

REFERENCES

American Occupational Therapy Association. (2008). Occupational therapy practice framework: Domain and process, 2nd edition. *American Journal of Occupational Therapy, 62*(6), 609–639.

Lin, C., & Browder, D. M. (1990). An application of engineering principles of motion study for the development of task analyses. *Education and Training in Mental Retardation , 25,* 367–375.

Miller, T. W., Ryan, M., & York, C. (2005). Using algorithms and pathways of care in allied health practice. Internet *Journal of Allied Health Sciences & Practice, 3*(2), 1–18.

Yuen, H. K., & D'Amico, M. (1998). Deriving directions through procedural task analysis. *Occupational Therapy in Health Care, 11,* 17–25.

Zemke, R., & Clark, F. (1996). *Occupational science: An evolving discipline.* Philadelphia, PA: F.A. Davis.

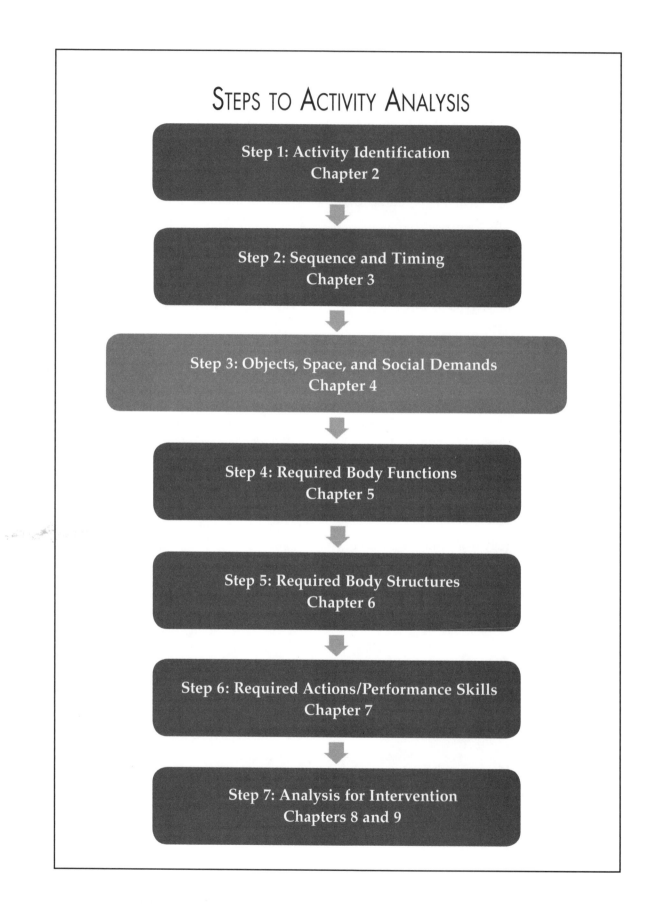

Steps to Activity Analysis

Step 1: Activity Identification
Chapter 2

Step 2: Sequence and Timing
Chapter 3

Step 3: Objects, Space, and Social Demands
Chapter 4

Step 4: Required Body Functions
Chapter 5

Step 5: Required Body Structures
Chapter 6

Step 6: Required Actions/Performance Skills
Chapter 7

Step 7: Analysis for Intervention
Chapters 8 and 9

4

OBJECTS, SPACE, AND SOCIAL DEMANDS

OBJECTIVES

1. Relate how frames of reference and ecological models shape our understanding of how the environment can influence participation in occupations and activities.

2. Understand how to determine the required equipment, tools, and materials for an activity or occupation.

3. Identify the properties of objects used during an activity and the influence these have on performance.

4. Define the space demands of activity and the impact on participation.

5. Understand how to determine the social demands of an activity and how they impact participation.

Once the steps and sequence of an activity are understood, the clinician must gain an understanding of the objects that are used during the activity and the particular properties of these objects. Understanding the objects and space required allows for a greater understanding of the skill and body functions that are required. For example, to fully understand the physical and cognitive demands of making a pine wood derby car, it is important to understand what materials and tools are used to make one. Information regarding properties of the wood used (how soft or hard the wood is) and the type of glue or paint that is used will help clarify the amount of strength, motor control, and other factors a person must have in order to make a derby car.

Understanding the objects that are required to perform an activity gives us another perspective on how the client will be interacting with his or her environment. Most physical (and cognitive) activities require that the person be doing something "with" something. Try to imagine an occupation that does not involve objects. Even simple activities such as walking or running require objects such as shoes. By gaining an understanding of what is used to perform the task, we can begin to look at what can be changed in order to allow for greater independence (covered in great detail in Chapter 9). For example, if we examine the occupation of self-feeding, the objects used include utensils, a table and chair, plate or bowl, cup, and, of course, food. If we are working with a client who has demonstrated difficulty with self-feeding, we will want to ensure that we not only look at what is occurring within the person that could be causing difficulty (such as decreased hand strength or range of motion) but also look at how we could change the objects used to allow for greater independence. Perhaps we can increase the size of the handles on the utensils to compensate for decreased hand strength.

In many of the models for occupational therapy (OT) practice such as the Person Environment Occupational Performance model (Christiansen & Baum, 1997), Ecology of Human Performance model (Dunn, Brown, & McGuigan, 1994), and the Person Environment model (Law et al., 1996), occupational performance is influenced by the interaction of elements within the person, the environment, and the occupation. Changes in any of these influence occupational performance. These models illustrate the need to thoroughly understand the occupation

Thomas, H. *Occupation-Based Activity Analysis* (pp. 49-57). © 2012 SLACK Incorporated

that the client is attempting to perform, so that the demands of the occupation (such as the objects) can be identified as a possible focus of intervention. These models are called *ecological* models in that they address the relationship between the human (all physical, mental, and spiritual aspects) and the physical and social environment (Brown, 2009). Part of the physical environment is the objects that we interact with while doing tasks or occupations. The influence of the social environment will be discussed in Chapter 8 in the discussion on contexts.

TOOLS

Tools used to perform an activity are objects such as scissors, pants, skis, or a stapler. While the most common image of a tool is one that might be used to do car repair or yard work, according to the *Cambridge Advanced Learner's Dictionary* (2009), a tool is defined as something that helps you complete an activity. Using a broader perspective on what a tool does and what it is used for allows us to think about how it applies to everyday occupations. What allows us to brush our teeth, comb our hair, or start our car every day? All of these are examples of occupations that require the use of tools. Tools are considered those objects that are not disposable and are reusable (they are not expendable like materials, which will be discussed in the next section). In the example of brushing teeth, the toothbrush would be considered the tool used, and the toothpaste is a material that is required.

MATERIALS

Material objects are physical articles that are needed to make or do something that become depleted during the process of the activity. One definition of *material* is that it is the substance or substances out of which things are made (*American Heritage Dictionary*, 2004). They could also be considered substances that are consumed or expended during the course of an activity. For example, writing materials would be the paper (which becomes used the moment it is written on) and the writing utensil, which expends ink or led, a material that cannot be reused (Figure 4-1). The *Occupational Therapy Practice Framework, 2nd Edition* (*Framework*) lists paint, milk, and lipstick as examples of materials (American Occupational Therapy Association [AOTA], 2008). It is important to recognize that materials are objects that may need to be replenished at the end of an activity or after a certain amount of time (as in the example of paint, the supply becomes diminished with each use). When

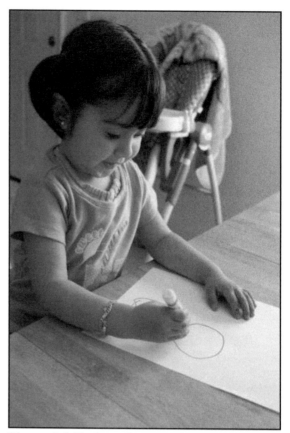

Figure 4-1. Tools and materials.

identifying the materials needed for an activity, it may be necessary to identify the amount needed (how much paint) and the properties of those materials and objects (type of paint). Properties will be discussed later in this chapter.

EQUIPMENT

In the case of activity analysis, *equipment* is defined as instruments or appliances that serve to equip someone to complete an activity (*Merriam-Webster Online Dictionary*, 2010). Equipment identified as required for an activity is often physically larger than the tools and may be considered a machine, such as a microwave or vacuum cleaner. Equipment can also be considered a set of objects that equip someone for a task, such as the hard hat, tool belt, kneepads, and gloves needed by a construction worker. The *Framework* uses workbench, stove, and basketball hoop as examples of equipment. It is often a challenge to distinguish between what is a tool and what is equipment. Tools are often manipulated or used by hand to assist in a task, while equipment tends to be larger or mechanical in nature. Technically, a piece of equipment can be used as a tool (an electric drill can be used to hang a picture). Whether you define an object as a tool or equipment is not essential, what is important is that you are able to identify all types of objects required of the activity, large, small, gas-powered, electric, or nonmotorized.

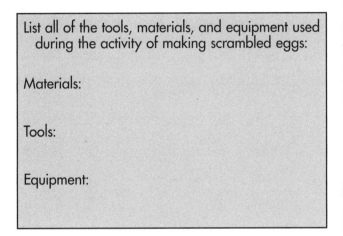

List all of the tools, materials, and equipment used during the activity of making scrambled eggs:

Materials:

Tools:

Equipment:

PROPERTIES

For many activities, the objects used must have certain inherent properties in order to allow for success in the activity. A *property* is an essential quality or distinctive trait of a physical object (*Merriam-Webster Online Dictionary*, 2010). The properties of an object are termed using descriptive words such as *red*, *heavy*, or *industrial strength*. Often a particular type of material or object is required, such as in a particular type of glue or paint. The properties of the objects used may be key to how the activity is conducted, time elements, and the skill set required. For example, *oil* is a term that is used to describe the property of a particular type of paint, which has characteristics that demand very different actions, skills, and time elements than a paint with a different property such as *water paints*.

The properties of objects needed for an activity as it is typically done are very different than those needed for an occupation that a particular person participates in. This is especially true in occupations when there is a variety in the types of supplies that could be used. For example, if you were to list the objects used to make a pine wood derby car, the tools used to carve and create the car may differ depending on the builder. To learn more about this occupation, I visited a derby car race held in Los Angeles. In my unofficial study of this occupation, I interviewed several of the racers and asked them about how they created their cars. Some of them purchased a kit, which contained a preshaped car, and some paint, and the builder used glue and other objects around the house to decorate it. Others chose to start from

scratch with a solid piece of wood and carve out the shape themselves. Even with this method, the tools used varied in that the type of knife used was dependent on the builder's experience and preference. This is where naming the specific properties of the objects used is of great utility. Not only is naming the properties important for some activities such as in cooking lobster (you need a large pot with a lid) but when conducting an occupation-based activity analysis for a particular client (understanding the particulars of the equipment, tools, and materials they prefer to use).

SPACE DEMANDS

Determining the space required of an activity requires examining the type of physical environment typically needed in order to perform the activity. The type of environment can range from an indoor area to requiring a wall of ice running down a cliff. The area used to perform an activity may need to be at a particular climate with specific temperature, humidity, or ventilation requirements. For most activities, these elements have little influence on performance, but for others, they are essential. For example, when painting the inside of a house, a certain amount of ventilation is required, the humidity cannot be too high or the paint will not dry, and it cannot be so cold that the paint freezes. The demands for certain temperature, ventilation, and humidity are strongly linked to the objects and properties used for the activity. Certain objects may become unusable in certain environments (such as snow in a hot environment) or may become unsafe (like the fumes of glue in an unventilated room).

Size

The size of the area needed is also an important aspect to determine. For example, if your client wants to race pine wood derby cars, how long is the track that the cars are raced on? This will determine how much space is required to participate in this activity. There may also be demands for a specific arrangement of the objects in the environment. Certain objects may need to be spaced a certain distance apart or above and below each other. For example, in the game of chess, the chess pieces need to be arranged in a certain way before the game can start. When we take a shower, the soap and shampoo must be arranged so that they are within reach while in the shower. Thinking about the arrangement of objects for an activity helps us in planning treatment sessions as well. If we know that certain objects need to be placed in a certain position, we can arrange for this to allow our clients greater success.

Arrangement of Objects in Space

It may be the arrangement and space required for the placement of objects that provides the challenge for our clients. We may mentally conduct an activity analysis on multiple activities to find an activity that has an arrangement that is "just right" within the space we are looking for. For example, if we were to try to find an activity that would challenge a client's ability to flex his shoulder above 90 degrees, we would want to find an activity that has objects that are placed above the head. Taking a shower curtain off to be washed would be an example of an activity in which the objects in the activity are placed in a position that would require a reach above 90 degrees of flexion (Figure 4-2). Finding activities that match not only what our client needs to improve upon but what they might actually do on a normal day is the challenge an OT practitioner is confronted with every day. Thus, our activity analysis skills become honed over time, further promoting OT's reputation as the activity analysis experts.

Surface

The surface required for an activity can range from a flat tabletop to rough pavement. As with all of the previous activity demands, the surface needed depends on the type of activity and the challenge you are seeking. Riding a bike can be done on many surfaces, but riding over rocks will be much more difficult than smooth pavement. For some activities, the type of surface is not an option. Writing with a pen and paper, for example, must be done on a hard, smooth surface to be successful. In order to downhill ski, the surface must be smooth and at a slight incline. In racing pine wood derby cars, the same is true; the surface must be smooth, without obstruction, and at an incline.

Lighting

The next space demand to consider is how much lighting is required and what type. For some activities, the type and amount of lighting is not particularly important (i.e., watching television). However, when reading or conducting activities that require a fine amount of visual acuity, the amount of light will influence success with the activity. When considering if lighting is important, ask yourself the following questions: Does the activity require visualizing fine details? Does the amount of light influence safety? Does lighting influence social interaction (e.g., with a singles' party)? Is lighting needed to establish a certain environment (such as for quiet meditation)? Answering these questions can start to uncover what lighting needs there may be for the activity you are analyzing. This is an area of the space

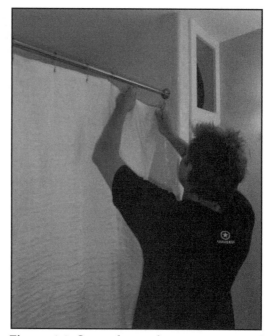

Figure 4-2. Space demands: arrangement of objects in space.

demands that can be easily overlooked to result in disaster. Several years ago, I planned a manicure group with several ladies who were patients at a hospital in which I worked. I set up a round table and carefully laid out all of the materials needed. However, when the ladies began to work on their nails, I found that the lighting in the room was dark and dingy, and several of the ladies were not able to see well enough to get the fingernail polish onto their nails correctly. Focusing only on the materials and surface needed, I missed a key ingredient to this activity.

The light that is inherent to the activity should also be considered, as this will influence the skills and client factors required to participate in the activity. The amount of light may fluctuate throughout the activity, requiring the eyes to accommodate to the change from bright to low lighting (such as in driving at night or at daytime and into a tunnel). The amount of light may be due to the nature of the activity, where there is either a low level of lighting (as in deep water scuba diving) or very bright lighting (such as in summer surfing). Of course, these levels of lighting are not required to complete the task but are a natural part of the activity.

Temperature

For most activities, having a certain temperature is not a requirement to complete the task. Having a comfortable temperature may be preferred by the patient or clinician, but it may not be required of the activity. So, when determining the temperature

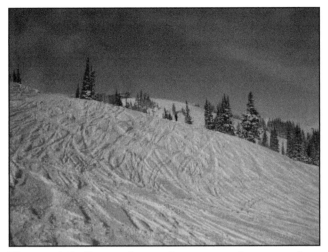

Figure 4-3. Space demands: temperature requirements of the environment.

requirements of the activity, think about what is absolutely necessary. For some activities, either heat or cold is needed, such as with Bikram's yoga, which is done in a studio that has been heated to 105 degrees Fahrenheit. This particular type of yoga is unique in that to be truly done successfully, the poses and movements must be done in extreme heat. Other activities, such as snow skiing, must be done in relatively cold weather, as the cold is what provides for the production and maintenance of the substance utilized to ski on: snow (Figure 4-3). It is often the objects utilized that determine the temperature required for an activity. Thus, when conducting an activity analysis, the objects and properties of the activity should be determined first.

When conducting an occupation-based activity analysis for a particular client, the temperature requirements may change, as you are determining what the temperature demands are for that particular person and in his or her contexts. For example, Pat has been an avid scuba diver her entire life. Over the last few years, she has been limited in her ability to perform many activities due to rheumatoid arthritis. She is now only able to scuba dive in warm water. Diving in cold water not only causes disabling pain in her joints, but putting on and taking off a wet suit causes strain on the joints in her fingers. Pat claims now that she is only a warm-water scuba diver. If conducting an activity analysis on this occupation for Pat, in order for her to be successful at the occupation, temperature would need to be considered a requirement of the activity.

Humidity

Just as with temperature, humidity level may be preferred by the client or clinician but may not always be a requirement. The objects utilized during the activity are often what determine the humidity needs for an activity. For example, painting the exterior of a house requires a lower level of humidity in order to allow the paint to dry. The key to determining level of humidity is to separate what is comfortable from what is essential. I am sure that those who live in areas of the world that experience very warm, humid summers would prefer to have lower humidity while conducting their everyday activities; however, it is not required for most people and activities. As with the example of Pat, where an occupation-based activity analysis found that she required a particular temperature to participate in her occupation, the same is true when determining the humidity requirements of occupation-based activity analyses; the demands for a particular person in their contexts may be different than the demands of the activity as it is typically done.

Noise

Noise, the type of noise, or the lack of noise is often a key factor to an activity. Imagine for a moment a high school prom with no music. The noise in this activity is music played loudly enough to facilitate dancing. In other situations, the lack of noise may be what is required. The activity of taking a test is an example of where the absence of sound is required for success in the activity. Typically, studying is an activity that might be considered an activity that requires quiet and minimal noise. However, if you conducted an occupation-based activity analysis with one of your classmates, you might find that he or she requires music in the background in order to study. This again shows how an occupation-based activity analysis may find different activity demands than those found in a standard activity analysis. When determining the noise requirements for a standard activity analysis, you will identify what the most common requirement for successful participation in the activity is.

The noise level that is inherent and produced by the activity should also be considered. Noises produced by equipment or people may not be required for success, but they are a necessary part of the activity. For example, the activity of vacuuming a rug includes the noise that the vacuum cleaner produces when running. When analyzing this activity, the amount of noise that is produced should be noted, as it may be a factor to consider when working with a client. For example, Hakima has a 14-year-old son, Neo, who has autism. He would like Neo to start taking on house chores, but he is hypersensitive to sounds and smells. In developing a list of chores with which Neo could help, you will want to analyze each as to the level of noise and smells they produce. Vacuuming would not be an activity that you would want to ascribe to him.

The level of noise that an activity produces influences the level of sensory ability required by the activity. An activity with a high level of noise requires a higher level of sensory processing ability. A lower level of noise may require a higher level of hearing ability. While taking a person's blood pressure, hearing a heartbeat through a stethoscope is required. This heartbeat is produced at a low volume level, demanding the participant to have a higher level of hearing ability.

It is important to also recognize and identify other elements of the activity that are instrumental to the demands of the activity and may impact performance. The environment in which the activity takes place or the objects utilized may generate sensations such as smell and touch. An odor may be emitted during part of the activity and may cue the participant to action (such as a burning smell when cooking) or may be part of the environment in which the activity is taking place and may require the participant to be able to endure the scent (such as the smell of cow manure while milking a cow).

Other features of the environment or objects used during the activity may create sensations of pressure or light touch on the skin. Some activities may cause the skin to be wet (scuba diving) or have other moist textures touching the skin (applying shaving cream or lotion to the skin). The texture of the environment may be rough or considered "scratchy," such as with building sand castles or walking barefoot in grass. When analyzing the environment and objects used in an activity, it is essential to identify possible sensory stimuli that may occur during the activity, as when analyzing the activity for a client, their sensory processing abilities will need to match the challenges presented during the activity.

Ventilation

According to the *Merriam-Webster Online Dictionary* (2010), *ventilation* is the circulation of air and the process of providing fresh air. When determining the amount of ventilation required of an activity, it will be important to understand the objects involved in the activity and the potential for emission of fumes, gasses, odors, and other elements that may become dangerous if inhaled. This is especially important when using chemicals, paint, or glue. Ventilation and the flow of air may be required to maintain a humidity level as well.

SOCIAL DEMANDS

When an activity occurs with other people, in the presence of others, or has an influence on others, social rules and expectations become part of the demands of an activity. Social rules are the typical norms and expectations of how one should act and communicate when involved in doing the activity. Depending on the activity, there may be expectations of behavior toward other people participating in the activity, such as how one responds to a question or to another person's actions. For other activities, the behavior expected may not involve acting or communicating toward another person but the actions or behaviors could influence another person. An example of this would be the social expectation that a person cooking food would wash their hands and not drop the food on the floor. For many everyday activities, there are unspoken social rules that are learned over time or as a child grows up. For example, in the activity of shopping, a social rule in most North American areas is that in order to make a purchase, one must wait in a line behind other shoppers who arrived to make their purchases first. This not a rule that is written down in a "shoppers instruction manual" but is part of most of the culture as a social expectation. When conducting an activity analysis of an activity as it is typically done, you will need to determine the social demands with the common culture. This may be difficult, as you will have to use your awareness of the activity, your observation skills of others performing the activity, and any written information you may find on the activity (if available). The social demands of an activity are important to identify, as the necessary social demands will assist us in detecting the required performance skills and body functions of the activity (Figure 4-4).

What are activities that typically require a high level of noise?

What are activities that typically produce a high level of noise?

What are activities that typically require a low level of noise?

What are activities that typically produce a low level of noise?

Other sensory features:

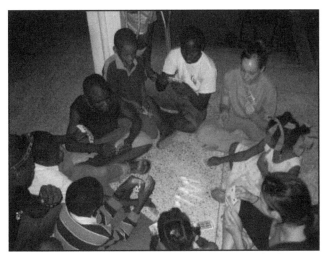

Figure 4-4. Social demands: occupational therapy students teach a game in Haiti.

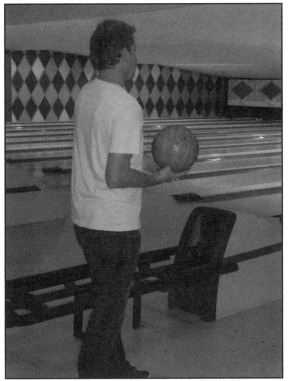

Figure 4-5. Social expectations: same activities may have different social demands.

Social rules and expectations are shaped and determined by the culture and social environment that the activity takes place in. Therefore, when determining the social demands of an activity, the environment in which the activity typically takes place must first be determined. Are there other people involved or within the space in which the activity occurs? The behavior and social communication styles expected while eating in other countries could be very different. In some cultures, it is rude to talk while eating, while in others it is expected. Some cultures expect that women and children eat after the men, while in others all people eat together.

Even activities that occur within the same country or culture can vary in the social demands depending on the social environment in which it occurs. Some social circles have roles and certain expectations of behavior from the members of their society. For example, a teen who enjoys the activity of bowling may have different social expectations when bowling with his or her friends (such as yelling and laughing at each other, giving each other "high-fives," and using words or terms not used with adults) than the social expectations when bowling with his or her parents (Figure 4-5). Understanding the different social contexts and various expectations will be important when conducting an occupation-based activity analysis. You will need to gain an awareness of your client's social roles and social contexts to help in determining the social demands of the activity. It is possible for a client to participate in the same activity but in several different contexts or social environments that require different social demands.

CONCLUSION

Gaining an understanding of the objects and environment utilized during an activity allows for greater perspective of the demands on the client's body functions and skill level. OT practitioners understand the relationship between the physical and social environment and participation in occupations. Just as a challenging physical environment, the social demands of an activity can influence engagement in an occupation, such as the rules of a game or the expectations of others. The tools, equipment, and materials also influence participation, as aspects such as size, shape, and complexity place demands on the client. Understanding how objects, space, and social demands play a role in an activity allows the clinician to develop strategies for adaptation and intervention.

Activity

Continue to analyze the activity of washing hair in the shower as it is typically done (not an occupation-based analysis on how you do it). Start by identifying which area of occupation it belongs to as well as which subcategory, followed by the objects and properties needed, space, and social demands. Include the sequence of steps you completed as part of Chapter 3. See Appendix A for full form.

1. Identify the activity or task:

Area(s) of occupation: Subcategory:

ADL

_____

IADL

_____

Education

_____

Work

_____

Play

_____

Leisure

_____

Social participation

_____

2. Objects and their properties:

3. Space demands:

4. Social demands:

5. Sequence and timing:

QUESTIONS

1. What is the difference between tools, materials, and equipment? Why is it important to identify each of these?

2. List at least five examples of properties of objects.

3. What aspects of the space demands must be determined for an activity analysis?

4. In what situations would it be important to have a specific temperature or ventilation?

5. What are the social demands of traveling by airplane?

REFERENCES

American Heritage dictionary of the English language (4th ed.). (2004). Boston, MA: Houghton Mifflin Company.

American Occupational Therapy Association. (2008). Occupational therapy practice framework: Domain and process (2nd ed.). *American Journal of Occupational Therapy, 62*(6), 609-639.

Brown, C. (2009). Ecological models in occupational therapy. In E. B. Crepeau, E. S. Cohn, & B. A. Boyt Schell (Eds.). *Willard & Spackman's occupational therapy* (11th ed., pp. 435–445). Philadelphia, PA: Lippincott Williams & Wilkins.

Cambridge advanced learner's dictionary (3rd ed.). (2009). Cambridge, UK: Cambridge University Press.

Christiansen, C., & Baum, C. (Eds.). (1997). *Occupational therapy: Enabling function and well-being* (2nd ed.). Thorofare, NJ: SLACK Incorporated.

Dunn, W., Brown, C., & McGuigan, A. (1994). The ecology of human performance: A framework for considering the impact of context. *American Journal of Occupational Therapy, 48,* 595–607.

Law, M., Cooper, B., Strong, S., Stewart, D., Rigby, P., & Lettes, L. (1996). The person–environment–occupation model: A transactive approach to occupational performance. *Canadian Journal of Occupational Therapy, 63,* 9–23.

Merriam-Webster online dictionary (2010). Merriam-Webster Online. Retrieved from http://www.merriam-webster.com/dictionary/equipment

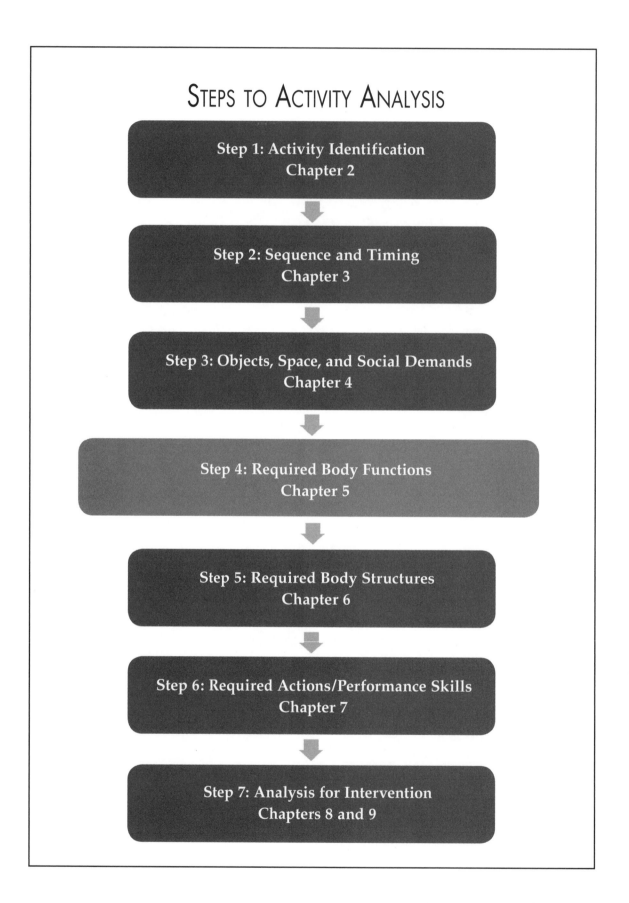

5

REQUIRED BODY FUNCTIONS

OBJECTIVES

1. Define body functions as they relate to client factors.

2. Describe how to determine the extent to which a body function is challenged during an activity.

3. Understand each of the mental function categories and how they are challenged and utilized during activities.

4. Define each of the sensory functions and how they are challenged and utilized during activities.

5. Understand each of the neuromusculoskeletal and movement-related functions and how they are utilized during performance of activities.

6. Describe each of the cardiovascular, hematological, immunological, and respiratory system functions and how they are challenged during participation in activities.

7. Identify each of the voice and speech functions and how they are challenged during participation in activities.

8. Define each of the digestive, metabolic, and endocrine functions as they relate to the demands of participation in an activity.

9. Understand each of the genitourinary and reproductive functions and how they are challenged during participation in activities.

10. Describe skin and related structure functions as they relate to the demands of participation in an activity.

Understanding the demands that an activity has for certain body functions requires examining the cognitive, physical, emotional, and sensory systems required. The *Occupational Therapy Practice Framework, 2nd Edition* (*Framework*) utilizes the *International Classification of Functioning, Disability and Health* (ICF) to define *body functions*: "the physiological functions of body systems (including psychological functions)" (World Health Organization [WHO], 2001, p. 10). Body functions are one part of the underlying client factors, or the "specific abilities, characteristics, or beliefs that reside within the client" (American Occupational Therapy Association [AOTA], 2008) p. 630). There are three aspects to client factors: (1) values, beliefs, and spirituality; (2) body functions; and (3) body structures (AOTA, 2008, p. 634). These client factors and the body functions are listed in Table 2 of the *Framework*. Conducting an activity analysis requires examining which of the body functions and body structures are required for the activity (see Table 3 of the *Framework*: Activity Demands).

Body functions are physiological aspects of the human body such as sensory, mental, neuromuscular, skeletal, and cardiovascular functions. For example, a function of the neuromuscular system is joint range of motion. In Table 2 of the *Framework*, body functions are listed according to categories, which are sometimes broken down into subcategories. For example, the broad category of mental functions is broken down into "specific mental functions" and "global mental functions." Each of these categories is further broken down into subcategories. Under "specific mental functions" there is a subcategory of "attention." Under this subcategory, specific body functions are listed: sustained, selective, and divided

Thomas, H. *Occupation-Based Activity Analysis* (pp. 59-105). © 2012 SLACK Incorporated

attention (AOTA, 2008). The body functions listed in the *Framework* are not intended to be an all-inclusive list but are designed to be a guide for clinicians in understanding the underlying body functions that influence participation in occupations (AOTA, 2008).

Client factors are the features that reside within the client that influence skill level but do not assure skill level needed to be successful in an activity (AOTA, 2008). A person's physical and mental well-being affects a person's skill and patterns but is also affected by external aspects such as the demands of the activity and the context in which it is performed. For example, a person may have a certain level of vestibular and muscle strength functions, but that does not assure that they will have the skill required to ski down an expert ski slope. Other demands of the activity influence successful performance in an occupation, such as the space demands (the level of incline of the ski slope) and the objects and properties used (the type of skis and boots used). As stated earlier, body functions and the other aspects of client factors can impact skill and success in an activity, especially if the body functions have been impaired by disease or illness. For example, a person with decreased muscle power will have difficulty maneuvering the skis around on the snow, and his or her skill level in this activity will be impaired.

An understanding of all of the steps required of the activity and what constitutes successful participation is needed to accurately identify all of the body functions demanded of the activity (and to what extent). All of the body function categories must be considered, as most activities challenge a variety of human factors. For example, in playing the game of tennis, not only are neuromusculoskeletal and movement-related functions used to run and hit the ball with a racket, but cardiovascular and respiratory systems are challenged, as well as mental and sensory functions, to see the ball and plan out a strategy to hit it. It is in determining the body factors required of an activity that the complexity of occupations is revealed. What might be considered a simple or everyday activity requires a complex combination of body functions, all working in conjunction.

When determining the body function demands of an activity, the occupational therapy (OT) practitioner must determine *to what extent* the presence or absence of a certain body function is required of the activity. In other words, how much is each body function challenged during the activity? The clinician must have an understanding of the physical, mental, and sensory challenges the activity has on the human body. This is where the method used for gathering information regarding each step of the activity (as discussed in Chapter 3) becomes so important. If a clinician is analyzing an activity in which he or she is not familiar and the steps of the activity are merely mentally visualized, the clinician may not correctly identify the key body functions needed to allow for full participation in the activity. To begin to understand how body functions relate to the demands of an activity, this chapter asks the reader to analyze activities by rating the extent to which each body function is challenged. A body function that is not utilized during the activity would be considered not challenged at all, and thus on the activity analysis sheet, "none" would be marked. A *minimal* challenge would be indicated when the body function is utilized but very minimally. A body function that is utilized to a large extent is one that is challenged to a *great* degree.

There may be times in which the extent to which a body function is required may be difficult to determine, as how much or how little a body is challenged is influenced by the contexts that surround it. Therefore, when conducting an activity analysis of how an activity is typically done, one must base the analysis on the context that is most common for that activity. Hypothetical situations or "what-if" scenarios should not be considered when trying to determine what body functions are required. For example, if analyzing the activity of making scrambled eggs, you would not include the body function of divided attention, because "maybe" the person has to also watch his or her children while making the scrambled eggs. Refrain from adding other elements within the context of the activity or adding other activities to the one you are analyzing. If conducting an occupation-based activity analysis, a full understanding of how the client typically conducts the activity, as well as the contexts in which it is performed, will need to be determined. The body functions required should be based on the list of steps you have already created in step 2 of the activity analysis, regardless of which type of analysis you are conducting. Using this as a guide will also eliminate the temptation to prematurely adapt the activity. For example, making scrambled eggs requires the use of both hands to crack each egg open. Yes, it can be adapted and done one-handed, but it is most commonly done with two hands.

ORGANIZATION OF THE BODY FUNCTION CATEGORIES

The *Framework* uses the ICF (WHO, 2001) classifications to organize the different body functions. There are eight broad categories:

1. Mental functions—Section 1

2. Sensory functions and pain—Section 2

3. Neuromusculoskeletal and movement-related functions—Section 3

4. Functions of cardiovascular, hematological, immunological, and respiratory systems—Section 4

5. Voice and speech functions—Section 5

6. Digestive, metabolic, and endocrine functions—Section 5

7. Genitourinary and reproductive functions—Section 5

8. Skin and related structure functions—Section 5

Within each of these broad categories, there may be subcategories. The subcategories may delineate and help further define the different aspects of the broad category. For example, mental functions are divided into either specific or global mental functions. Under each of these lie subcategories that further define each of the two areas. For example, under specific mental functions, there are eight subcategories: higher level cognitive, attention, memory, perception, thought, sequencing complex movement, emotional, and experience of self and time. These are not body functions but categories or groups of body functions. Under each of these categories are common body functions, such as short-term, long-term, and working memory—all body functions under the category of memory.

SECTION 1: MENTAL FUNCTIONS

Specific Mental Functions

Higher-Level Cognitive

There are seven specific higher-level cognitive functions listed in the *Framework*: judgment, concept formation, metacognition, cognitive flexibility, insight, attention, and awareness. Higher-level cognitive functions are often called *executive functioning*, which includes complex decision making, planning, and abstract thinking. All of these functions are controlled by the frontal lobes of the brain (WHO, 2001). These higher level cognitive functions allow us as humans to adapt to situations, think abstractly, and plan for the future. This category of functions is appropriately named higher level in that the thought processes exercised within these functions are not basic but are complex in nature.

Judgment

Judgment requires mentally examining the aspects of different options and discriminating the variation in order to form an opinion or belief. We utilize judgment throughout our day, weighing options in order to make good decisions. Judgment is a difficult skill to learn but is closely linked to utilizing past experiences and knowledge in order to understand the implications of each situation or option. In order to form an opinion, one must speculate the outcome and impact on not only themselves but others. For example, if a person decides to answer his cell phone while watching a movie in a theater, this might be seen as poor judgment, as it has an impact on others sitting in the theater. However, if the person's wife is pregnant and is expecting the baby at any time, the person needs make a judgment call, which is a subjective decision based on the information available. This man must quickly weigh the implications on himself and on others if he (a) answers the phone or (b) does not answer the phone.

When analyzing whether or not judgment is required of an activity, ask yourself the following questions: Does the activity require the person to form an opinion? Is the person required to weigh options? Does the activity require he or she understand the implications of each option? How much does this activity challenge his or her ability to make good judgments?

Real-world example: Mariem is 86 years old and lives in an assisted-living facility. Yesterday, she got a call from a "nice young man" who said that she had just won a drawing for a free trip to Hawaii. In order to process her prize, he needed her credit card number and social security number. Mariem found out the next day that her credit card had been charged to the limit and a new one opened up under her social security number. While reporting this to her credit card company, she admits that this was poor judgment on her part. What information should Mariem have gathered before making the decision to give the caller her information? What else may have contributed to utilizing good judgment in this case?

Concept Formation

Concept formation is the ability to organize information and develop ideas based on the common qualities of objects or situations. Concept formation is linking pieces of information or sensory experiences to form an understanding of something that is not concrete. It requires being able to define how objects and ideas are different and understand how certain concepts or objects are related (Zoltan, 2007). Concept formation is closely tied to abstraction and generalization. Abstraction is mentally processing and coordinating ideas that are outside of concrete instances. Abstract thought is used to understand and apply theories and intangible concepts. For example, to understand the concept of love one must link together notions of trust, caring, selflessness, and other nontangible concepts to create a concept of what love is and how this invisible feature of emotion and action evidences itself. Each person has a different concept of what love is based on his or her experiences.

To determine if concept formation is challenged during an activity, ask yourself the following questions: Does the activity require the person to mentally form concepts? Does the person need to mentally organize a variety of information to form theories or ideas? Does the activity require the person to understand abstract concepts (things that are not concrete)? Does the activity require that the person understand logical relationships between ideas (e.g., roosters and dolphins are animals), yet also understand differences? Does the person need to understand opposites (e.g., small instead of large)?

Metacognition

Metacognition is having an awareness of one's own cognitive processes and the ability to manipulate and control his or her own cognition (Zoltan, 2007). This is self-awareness of one's cognitive ability and is often defined as *thinking about thinking* (Brown, 1978). It is utilized to analyze a problem, monitor progress toward a solution, and in planning strategies toward the problem (Flavell, 1979). Metacognition is important for effective learning, problem solving, and for efficient communication with others (Al-Hilawani, 2003). Al-Hilawani measured metacognition by asking students to look at five pictures that each gave a different situation. The students were asked to sort out the pictures to find the one that did not fit the rest. While sorting through the pictures, the students were asked to verbalize how they were working through the problem. The researchers were examining each of the students' methods for obtaining and utilizing knowledge (Al-Hilawani, 2003). OT research and literature emphasizes the importance of metacognition on utilizing learning strategies, gaining an understanding how one best learns and retains information (Munguba, Valdes, & Da Silva, 2008). Metacognition emphasizes the use of all of the other aspects of cognitive functions such as judgment, memory, insight, awareness, recognition, and discrimination (Al-Hilawani, Easterbrooks, & Marchant, 2002).

Activities that require metacognition are those that require learning new information (creating strategies for learning and retaining the information), as well as activities that require sorting and organizing information. When analyzing an activity for the level

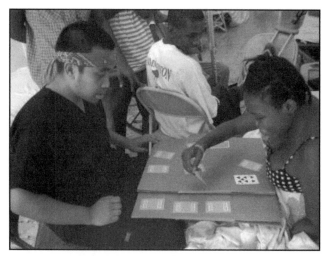

Figure 5-1. Cognitive flexibility: occupational therapy student using cardboard to create a table in Haiti.

of metacognition required, ask yourself if the activity requires that they have an understanding of their cognitive abilities. Does the activity require that they analyze a problem, create strategies for how they are going to solve the problem and be able to monitor how those strategies are working?

Cognitive Flexibility

Having cognitive flexibility requires changing strategies when confronting a problem, or changing a set of thoughts (WHO, 2001). This means that when presented with two or more concepts, the person can shift from one to the other. When presented with new information, a new opinion or approach can be formed as needed for the situation. To get a better understanding of this, it might be easier to think of what it means to be cognitively inflexible. You may have met someone who was inflexible in their acceptance of a concept or idea, despite how much you tried to inform them. People with difficulty in cognitive flexibility have difficulty changing strategies when there are changes in a situation or if there is an error (Parker, 1990). Therefore, when thinking about an activity and determining if cognitive flexibility is required, think about whether the activity requires the person to shift his or her thoughts as information is presented (Figure 5-1). Does the activity have the potential for error and require the person to change strategies? Does the activity require that the person shift from one idea to another?

Real-world example: Mary and John are out on their first date. They decide that they want to see the new romantic comedy movie that was just released and then have dinner afterward. When they arrive at the movie theater, they find out that all of the tickets for the movie have been sold out for the early evening show. There are only tickets available for the

8:30 show. Mary is incredibly disappointed. However, John decides that they can go to dinner first and then go to the movie afterward at 8:30. John's ability to change his plans based on the information presented demonstrates good cognitive flexibility.

Insight and Awareness

According to the ICF and most OT literature, insight is related to self-awareness and having an understanding on one's strengths and weaknesses (WHO, 2001; Zoltan, 2007). This means having a realistic concept of one's physical and mental capabilities. Insight into one's abilities is required in order to make safe decisions and to correct errors when they are made. This is also essential to adapting to problems as they may arise or adapting to a disability (why use a walker when they believe they can walk just fine?). Insight is also closely linked to judgment, as having poor insight into one's abilities may lead to poor decision making and judgments. Insight is required for goal setting and in establishing future plans.

According to Barco, Grosson, Bolesta, Werts, and Stout (1991) and Crosson et al. (1989), there are three types of awareness that influence participation in activities: intellectual, emergent, and anticipatory. Intellectual awareness is the ability to understand what abilities and weaknesses are present before engaging in the activity. With intellectual awareness, the person is able to verbalize any deficits that he or she may have. This is foundational for the other two types of awareness, in that without intellectual awareness, emergent and anticipatory awareness are limited. *Emergent awareness* occurs when the person is able to recognize limitations or strengths while they are occurring. *Anticipatory awareness* is the ability to predict or accept that a deficit will inhibit success or cause a problem (Barco et al., 1991). For example, a person may anticipate that he or she will not be able to climb the stairs leading up to the Lincoln Memorial based on his or her understanding of his or her abilities.

Awareness is necessary for activities that require advanced planning and use of specific skills. When determining if awareness or insight is required of an activity, ask yourself if the activity requires having an understanding of what one's strengths are. Does it require that the person be able to clearly understand what his or her weaknesses are? Does it require that he or she adapt tasks based on his or her weaknesses? Does the activity require setting personal goals? Does the activity require planning future events or achievements?

Real-world example: Dustin was out skiing with his buddies. At the end of the day, his buddies decided that they were going to ski the last run down an expert slope through a canyon. Dustin was not an expert skier, and he was very tired from a full day of skiing. Being aware of his current skiing ability, he decided not to join them on the last run and took an easier route down. This self-awareness and insight possibly saved Dustin from injury as he might have hurt himself trying to go down a slope that did not match his skill level.

Attention

Sustained Attention

Sustained attention requires maintaining concentration on one activity or stimulus for a sustained amount of time (WHO, 2001). Attention is focusing in on sensory information, choosing to process certain aspects of our environment or sensations. Thus, targeting our attention allows us to receive information, which also supports retention of information into memory (Zoltan, 2007). Sustaining attention requires vigilance toward maintaining thought and receiving sensory information. In determining if sustained attention is required of the activity you are analyzing, think about how long the person must sustain his or her focus on what is occurring. To what extent does the person have to focus? Are there opportunities for breaks or is continued focus required? An example of an activity that requires sustained attention is taking the National Board for Certification in Occupational Therapy (NBCOT) exam.

Selective Attention

Selective attention is focusing in on one or more stimuli, while all other stimuli or information in the environment are ignored (Zoltan, 2007). Selective attention requires actively discriminating between what information and stimulus to absorb and what to disregard. The demand for selective attention increases as the amount of external stimuli increases. The greater the intensity of the distracter, the greater the demand for selective attention will be. For example, many husbands and wives feel that their spouses have selective attention when watching their favorite TV show or football game, as they tend to not hear them when called. We may exercise selective attention when trying to study or read in a very noisy environment like an airport, where we need to filter out the noise and commotion around us to focus attention on what is being read. When determining if selective attention is required of an activity, determine how much external distracters there typically are during the activity. Where does the activity typically take place? Does the activity require that the person ignore other stimuli while focusing on one stimulus or a certain group of stimuli?

Divided Attention

Divided attention is utilized when a person must focus on two or more stimuli at one time (WHO, 2001). Activities such as cooking utilize divided attention, in that while focusing on chopping vegetables, one might also be attending to a pot of boiling water. Parents often become experts at divided attention, as they are constantly watching what their children are doing while trying to complete other tasks around the home. Divided attention is what allows us to do several tasks at once (Zoltan, 2007). It may require us to divide attention between different motor movements, cognitive processes, or both. For example, talking on the phone and driving requires divided attention between two different sets of motor movements, cognitive processes, and sensory stimulation. In order to successfully do both, we must attend to both what we hear on the phone and say to the person as well as what we see on the road and appropriately respond physically (turn the wheel or push the brake).

Memory

Memory is closely linked to other cognitive and sensory factors, in that the brain stores information on sensory experiences (Zoltan, 2007). A person must attend to a sensory experience, such as looking at a flower, before it can be encoded into memory. If a person does not experience something through visually hearing it, seeing it, or feeling it, he or she will not be able to recall it from memory (e.g., one does not recall what a manatee is if he or she has never heard or seen what one is). It is theorized that memories created out of sensations (sensory memory) are usually short term and are stored according to the type of input (auditory, visual, and tactile). It is from this short-term memory that information continues on into working memory or long-term memory (Zoltan, 2007).

Short-Term Memory

The memory function that produces storage of information temporarily, for about 30 seconds, is considered short-term memory. If not stored in long-term memory, this information is usually lost (WHO, 2001). Short-term memory is very limited, and is different than working memory (see next). It is what allows us to recall small chunks or bits of information for immediate use. For example, if you were to look up a phone number you might look at the phone number (or parts of it) and temporarily store it in your short-term memory long enough to dial the number on your phone. When determining if short-term memory is required of an activity, you will first need to determine if it is working memory or short-term memory that is needed. Short-term memory is used for small pieces of information that are used briefly.

It may be used to allow a person to move on to the next step of an activity (did I look both ways before crossing the street?). It is possible for an activity to require short-term memory as well as working memory.

Working Memory

Working memory is information that is retained while we are using it during a task (L. Levy, 2005). It is also understood to be temporary memory that allows for manipulation of information (Zoltan, 2007). It is working memory that allows us to hold information and use it during tasks. It is theorized that our working memory can handle seven pieces of information at one time (Parente & Anderson, 1991). We utilize working memory throughout our daily activities, such as when writing a letter, manipulating information and memories to write each sentence that links to the paragraph and paragraphs that complete a letter. In this example, the person writing the letter can go back and read what he or she has already written, which would be an inefficient way of completing the task. It is working memory that allows us to problem solve and process tasks that do not involve physical cues to the information (Zoltan, 2007). For example, when asked a question in class, students may utilize working memory to mentally think through the question, and store information regarding other students' answers, all to come up with their own answer. It is working memory that allows us to perform many of our everyday tasks that require a temporary hold of information for use in various aspects of the activity. Working memory might be used in order to create a strategy in a game by being able to recall an opponent's moves and actions.

When determining if working memory is required of an activity, look through the steps required and decide if any of these steps require mental manipulation of different pieces of information. (You will actually be using working memory to do this.) Does the activity require the person to recall and utilize chunks of information temporarily (these are not intended to be long-term memories). Does the activity require that he or she utilizes memories to guide actions? Does the activity require complex problem solving?

Long-Term Memory

Information about past events, language, and sensory experiences that are stored for long periods of time is part of the long-term memory system (WHO, 2001). These memories are retained for a few hours up to years (Zoltan, 2007). This allows for utilization of past experiences to deal with current ones. Information that is used during working memory is

Activity 5-1

REVIEW OF HIGHER LEVEL COGNITIVE FUNCTIONS

Identify how each of the following functions are utilized while buying a snack out of a vending machine (Figure 5-2). Assume that you are already standing in front of the machine with change in your pants pocket. Leave a row blank if a factor not used. In the final columns, indicate the extent to which each body function is challenged during this activity.

Function	How It Is Used	None	Minimally Challenged	Greatly Challenged
Judgment				
Concept formation				
Metacognition				
Cognitive flexibility				
Insight/ awareness				
Sustained attention				
Selective attention				
Divided attention				
Short-term memory				
Working memory				
Long-term memory				

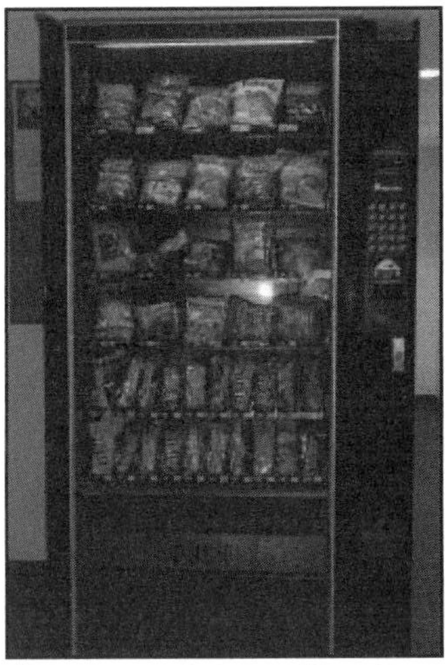

Figure 5-2. Vending machine.

retained and encoded into long-term memory. Thus, information that is rehearsed or utilized as working memory is more efficiently stored long term (Zemke, 1994). An example of long-term memory is recalling how to ride a bike, even after years of not having done this activity. We utilize long-term memory for activities that are repeated on a daily basis, such as brushing our teeth and driving home. Long-term memories are used for activities that require the ability to recall personal information (such as birth date and social security number), events (such as where you were yesterday at noon), facts (such as who the president is), and procedures (such as how to complete a task). When determining if an activity requires long-term memory, think about how far back they must remember (Activity 5-1). Do they need to remember events or information from over an hour ago? Do they need to recall how to do something they had done in the past? Do they need to be able to recall personal history?

Real-world example: Judi was attending a workshop where the speaker was using a VHS tape for her presentation. During the presentation, the tape became entangled in the player, causing the tape to break. The speaker was in a panic. Judi helped the speaker remove the tape and to her surprise was able to help. Judi's first job while in high school was working at a video rental store. Surprisingly, Judi was able to recall how to repair the VHS tape, a task she repeatedly conducted during her job at the rental store. This was a surprise to Judi, as this was not a skill she ever intended to use again and was amazed when her repair job allowed the tape to run again.

Perception

Discrimination of Sensations: Auditory Perception

Auditory perception allows for the ability to discriminate between different sounds, tones, and pitches (WHO, 2001). This is what allows us to differentiate between the sound of a refrigerator running and rain hitting the pavement outside. Perception of sound is different from the ability of the ear to transmit sound. Perception of sound relies on the brain to interpret signals sent from the ear about auditory information occurring in the environment. It is what allows us to understand an alerting noise (a scream) from a loud radio. This is not to be confused with *auditory memory*, which is the ability to remember what certain environmental stimuli sound like (such as remembering the sound of a good friend's voice). Auditory perception is utilized for tasks that require a person to distinguish between two or more different noises. It is required when the activity requires the person to take action based on a certain sound (such as with a fire alarm or ringing phone). Discrimination of different tones and pitches is used when communicating, singing, or playing musical instruments. Being able to discriminate between tones, pitches, and types of sounds is essential for interpreting much of what occurs in the environment (watch a movie on mute and see how much is missed or can be misunderstood). Different tones may help in determining where an activity is occurring or how. For example, a mother may listen at the doorway of the bathroom to determine if her child is truly in the bathtub washing or simply sitting outside of the tub, swishing the water around with his or her hand.

When determining if discrimination of auditory information is required of an activity, think about what actions are demanded of the person during the activity, not what ambient noise occurs during the activity. If discrimination of auditory information is required, the person engaged in the activity will be required to react or make decisions based on the sounds made in the environment. Does the ability to discriminate between sounds contribute to the person's ability to engage in the activity, or can it be done without? For example, attending a musical concert requires this function, while taking a shower does not. Both include noise, but taking a shower does not require the person to utilize the ability to discriminate or understand the noise made during the activity.

Discrimination of Sensations: Tactile

Tactile discrimination allows us to distinguish different textures by touch (WHO, 2001). It is our ability to perceive the difference in textures, not just the body's ability to sense touch (which will be addressed later in the sensory functions). Tactile discrimination is a perceptual function that gives us the ability to understand dimensions and physical characteristics of objects and determine if something is smooth or rough by touching it with some part

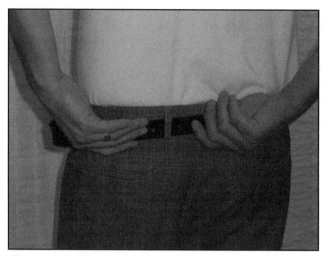

Figure 5-3. Discrimination of sensations: tactile.

of our body. Notice that this is under the category of "specific mental functions" because this function relies on the brain to interpret what is being felt.

Because we have a greater number of touch receptors in our fingers, humans tend to use their hands to "feel" or touch objects (Cooper & Abrams, 2006). Thus, when we use our hands (or feet) to complete tasks, we may be using our sense of touch to give us information about performance. This is especially true when aspects of the activity are conducted out of sight or information cannot be gathered through sight alone. For example, when stringing a belt through the belt loops of pants, a person must feel for the loops with his or her fingers and use the sense of touch to feel for the belt in order to pull it through (Figure 5-3). If the pants, the loops, and the belt all felt the same, the task would be very difficult to complete. Think about what allows you to put your hands in your purse of backpack and find an object without looking. Tactile discrimination is what allows us to process what we are feeling and understand the difference between two very similar objects such as a pen and a pencil.

Tactile discrimination is required of an activity if the person engaging in the activity must discriminate between different textures, such as smooth or rough, oily or dry, sticky or smooth. It may also be required if aspects of the activity are done without the use of sight. Think about some of the daily activities you do that use your sense of touch: shampooing your hair (feel if there are soap suds left), typing (feeling for the keys), buttoning buttons, or turning pages of a book.

Discrimination of Sensations: Visual

Visual discrimination is our ability to perceive and interpret visual information. It is what allows us to discriminate between different shapes, objects, and colors (WHO, 2001). It is important to distinguish

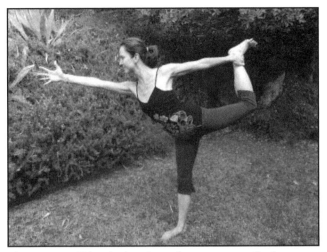

Figure 5-4. Discrimination of senses: vestibular-proprioception is used in great amounts in yoga.

the difference between visual discrimination as a perceptual function and vision as a sensory function. *Visual perception* is the cognitive processing of what our eyes detect. A person may have perfect oculomotor skill and intact eye structures and yet can be unable to perceive or understand what they see. Often referred to as *form discrimination* in the literature on visual perception, visual discrimination is primarily utilized to distinguish shape but also serves to distinguish and identify color, orientation, and edge (Zoltan, 2007). This is what allows us to react to the environment and interact with objects and people. Visual perception is required for a large majority of our everyday activities and works in conjunction with many other body functions for basic tasks such as standing or sitting upright or reaching for an object (Zoltan, 2007). To give you an example of how this function is used, set this book down, get up and go to the bathroom (yes, even if you don't have to go). As you travel, think about how you understand what you are seeing and what allows you to take the correct path and use the correct objects.

Are you back? To complete this activity, you used your visual discrimination skills to set your book down on a solid surface (it is this function that tells you where to place a book so it is not hanging off the edge of a table), to get up and walk toward a doorway or hallway and center your body as to not hit anything, identify which is a bathroom, place your hands on the door and push or pull as you see is needed, and visually identify how to walk in. How did you know which object was the toilet? How did you tell the difference between the toilet paper and a towel? (Hopefully you chose the correct one.) So much of what we do every day utilizes this ability to discriminate between objects, shapes, and colors.

Discrimination of Sensations: Olfactory

The use of olfactory discrimination is what allows for distinguishing differences in smells (WHO, 2001). It is what might alert us to a smell that requires action, such as smoke or fumes. It may be used to be able to identify if something is rotten (such as smelling a carton of milk after its expiration date to determine if it is still edible). Many parents use olfactory discrimination to determine if their child needs a diaper changed or if their teenage son needs to take a shower. There are many activities that involve the presence of smells, but when determining if olfactory discrimination is required, you must determine if participation in the activity requires that the person engaging in the activity must use this function in order to perform that activity. Does the activity require that the person act upon certain smells? Does the person need to be able to detect the absence or presence of certain aspects, such as if there are fumes from paint or glue in the air and ventilation is needed.

Discrimination of Sensations: Vestibular-Proprioception

The interaction between proprioception and vestibular perception influences positioning of the body in space. This is what allows us to determine how to hold ourselves upright or in a certain position for an activity (de Bruin, 2008). Perception of vestibular input is what tells us what direction we are moving in, the speed of our movement, our head position, and the position of our body in space (WHO, 2001). This requires mentally processing the positional signals sent from the inner ear that indicate position of the head. Proprioception is detecting muscle lengthening, shortening, and how fast and in which direction a limb or body part is moving. It is together that vestibular and proprioceptive perception allows us to understand where our head and body parts are in relation to one another. This body function entails the interaction of the two to create a perception of where one's body is in space (Figure 5-4).

To determine if this function is required of an activity, think about what positions or positional changes occur during the activity. Does the activity require that the participant bend over and then come to an upright position again? Does the activity require that the person understand and regulate how quickly his or her body is moving? Does he or she need to be able to position his or her body in a certain direction? Does the position of his or her head change during the activity? Is vision occluded or limited and thus the person must position him- or herself based on vestibular and proprioceptive sense instead of by sight? An example of this is dancing, where body parts are moving outside of sight, position of the head may rotate, the dance may require leaning to one side bending down but then coming back to an upright position. This perceptual ability contributes greatly to balance as well.

Multisensory Processing

Multisensory processing is the integration of sensory information from different sources (auditory, vestibular, touch, olfactory, proprioceptive functions) to better interpret what is occurring in the environment (Roley & Jacobs, 2009). To gain an understanding of objects or our environment, we utilize a variety of senses. Multisensory processing is a mental function that allows us to utilize this information together. For example, during the activity of washing our hair in the shower, we utilize our sense of touch, temperature, proprioception, and vestibular perception to understand the sensations occurring during the activity and what they mean in regards to how we should react.

When determining if multisensory processing is required of an activity, think about what different sensations must be processed and understood during the activity. Are there sensations that occur simultaneously? Are multiple sensations utilized to understand aspects of an activity? For example, while typing these words on my computer, I am using my sense of touch to find the keys, auditory processing to hear that each press of the key was accepted, and visual discrimination to see what comes up on the screen as a result of my pressing the keys. All of this information is processed and integrated together to help me progress through the activity.

Sensory Memory

Sensory memory is the first stage of memory, which is the processing and brief storage of sensory input. It is very short term and is specific to the type of sensation (auditory, touch, etc.) (Zoltan, 2007). This allows us to hold a sensation in our memory briefly so that it can be processed. It is from sensory memory that we work with it in our working memory, and store it in short-term or long-term memory. We utilize sensory memory to understand a series of sensations. For example, we may need to briefly remember what we just saw in a movie picture frame to understand what occurs next. We retain visual information about what we saw in order to process and understand the next picture. Auditory information works in much the same way. When you are listening to an instructor lecture, you are momentarily storing each word he or she says to make sense of the sentence that is the end result. That sentence may then be stored in short-term memory or long-term memory depending on its use.

Sensory memory is utilized in almost all daily activities. If interacting with the environment, objects,

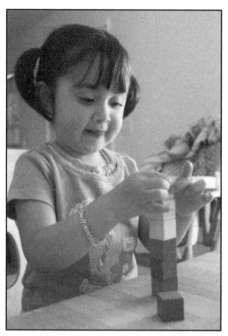

Figure 5-5. Spatial relationships.

or other people, some degree of sensory memory will be utilized. It is used if one visual image leads to another or one auditory piece of information leads to another (such as listening to someone talk or listening to a song). A tactile sensation may be temporarily stored in order to create a response, such as when a fly lands on your arm, you may quickly go to slap it, using your sensory memory to recall where it was on your arm.

Spatial Relationships

Also called *visuospatial processing*, the *spatial relationship function* is the ability to understand the position of objects in relation to you and between different objects (Figure 5-5). It is understanding and accurately interpreting distance, position, and orientation of objects and distinguishing objects from others surrounding it or in the background (Zoltan, 2007). This is what allows us to understand how far apart or close objects are. It is also used in basic tasks such as dressing (understanding what is the front and back of pants). This would be used when writing a letter, aligning each letter next to the next appropriately so that it creates a word and forming each word so that they fit on the page.

In determining if spatial relations is a function required of an activity, first think of the environment in which the activity occurs. Does it take place in a space in which the person participating in the activity will need to understand the distance between him or herself and objects? Will he or she be moving in relation to the objects or elements of the environment?

Activity 5-2

REVIEW OF PERCEPTION FUNCTIONS

Identify how each of the following functions is utilized while buying a snack out of a vending machine. Assume that you are already standing in front of the machine with change in your pants pocket. Leave a row blank if a factor is not used. In the final columns, indicate the extent to which each body function is challenged during this activity.

Function	*How It Is Used*	*None*	*Minimally Challenged*	*Greatly Challenged*
Discrimination of senses: Auditory				
Discrimination of senses: Tactile				
Discrimination of senses: Visual				
Discrimination of senses: Olfactory				
Discrimination of senses: Vestibular-proprioception				
Multisensory processing				
Sensory memory				
Spatial relationships				
Temporal relationships				

Will he or she need to manipulate objects? Does he or she need to perceive which is the top or bottom of an object? Does the activity require that he or she recognize an object separate from a background (e.g., see a shirt laying on a bed).

Temporal Relationships

The temporal relations function addresses the perception of and the passage of time (Levy & Dreier, 1997). This relates to the ability to have some internal sense of the duration or rate of a stimulus without the use of a clock, as well as understanding the relationship between what is seen, heard, and felt and timing (Shams, Kamitani, & Shimojo, 2004). During many activities, both sound and visual stimuli are produced at the same time in which perception of temporal relationships allows for an understanding that they are occurring at the same time. Understanding this "temporal synchronicity" allows us to understand that multiple sensory stimuli may occur from one action or element within our environment, creating sensory redundancy such that auditory information may support or correspond to what we see (Pizur-Barnekow, Kraemer, & Winters, 2008). For example, we may see a bouncing ball but also hear it bounce off the floor. It should be noted that despite the similar term used, this function is not related to the temporal lobe of the brain.

To determine if this perceptual function is required, think about if a concept of the passage of time is necessary for continuation on steps or discontinuation of steps. An example is understanding how long to brush teeth before stopping. Think also of the different sensory experiences that occur during the activity. Does the activity require the person to understand the timing of these different sensory experiences to understand what is occurring? Are there two or more sensory modalities present for one action (e.g., clapping hands provides tactile and auditory stimuli at the same time)? Does the activity require action that requires an understanding of timing, perception of the passing of time, rhythm, or pacing? Examples of this are answering the phone, playing a musical instrument, and walking across a street.

Use Activity 5-2 as a review for this section.

Thought Functions

Recognition

Using information from the environment to understand what is occurring requires recognition. We must recognize what we see, hear, and feel and be able to interpret what each means (Rahman & Sommer, 2008). If an orange is placed in front of us, we must be able to identify this as a food and not a ball to bounce on the floor. This applies to auditory information as well. We can recognize a car horn or the sound of a friend's footsteps. Using our ability to recognize objects, sounds, and textures is what allows us to act and engage during activities (Figure 5-6). We recognize words when reading or listening to someone speak. We recognize the shampoo bottle when in the shower and washing our hair. Many researchers argue that recognition is tied to memory and perceptual ability (Rahman & Sommer, 2008). This argument holds that prior exposure to an object or sound is stored in memory and is recalled when used to recognize stimuli. As with many of the other body functions, recognition does rely on operation of other functions in the sensory and perceptual categories in order to perform. Without the ability to see or perceive visual information, a person will have difficulty recognizing objects visually.

Recognition is required if interacting with objects and sounds or within an environment. Activities that involve other people require recognition of faces, actions, words spoken, and expressions. When analyzing an activity to determine if recognition is required, think about what objects are involved. Does the person engaging in the activity need to be able to recognize these objects and understand what they are? Does he or she need to be able to recognize aspects within an environment, such as a window, a door, or a curb on the street? Does the person need to be able to recognize language or sounds? Keep in mind that although sensory information may be present during an activity, you need to determine if the activity requires that he or she recognize the sensory information.

Categorization

Categorization is finding similarities and differences and putting objects or information into groups (Zoltan, 2007). This body function also relies on perceptual and sensory functions. Information is often categorized based on sensory features, such as certain physical features or types of sounds. Some categorization occurs based on symbolic characteristics or by functioning. For example, a bus, train, and bike can all be categorized as modes of transportation. Objects may also be categorized based

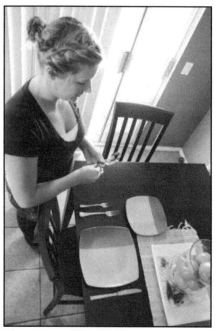

Figure 5-6. Recognition and categorization: setting the table.

on other traits such as weight, texture, or movement. For example, if a client is told he or she needs to eat soft foods, he or she needs to be able to categorize several food items that would be considered soft.

When determining if this thought function is used during an activity, it is again important to have a good understanding of what objects are used during the activity and what other sensory information will be presented during the activity. Does the activity require that the person understand the similarities between two or more objects? For example, when putting dishes away from the dishwasher, the different size dishes will be categorized into one area to be stored, while the cups will be grouped together in another. Another example would be when grocery shopping. Similar items such as cheese, milk, and yogurt can be mentally categorized based on the fact that they are all dairy items and will be located in the same area of the grocery store. Our ability to categorize is what shapes our actions and often determines success or struggle during an activity (Figure 5-7).

Generalization

Generalization is the ability to take a strategy learned in one situation and transfer it to a new or different situation or environment (Zoltan, 2007). Thus, what one is able to do in one setting will be generalized to other settings. For example, when a child learns to use a toilet to go to the bathroom, it may take a while for him or her to generalize or learn how to use that skill in other restrooms. As adults,

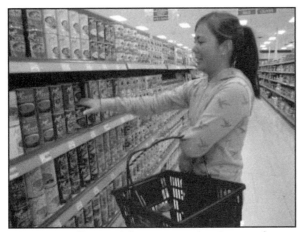

Figure 5-7. Recognition, categorization, and generalization: shopping.

we use generalization in many different aspects of life. If you were to rent a car, would you still be able to drive? Of course, as the skills you learned in your own car can be transferred over to this new context. Generalization is an important task when related to conducting parts or elements of an activity and how it is related to a larger task. For example, a client who buttons up a shirt that is sitting on his lap will need to understand that this is a task that is part of the activity of donning a shirt. Out of context, it may not make sense if he is limited in his ability to generalize. You will need to generalize the concepts you learn from reading this book to what you will do as a clinician.

To identify if generalization is required of an activity, think about the different settings that this activity is typically done in—is it now occurring in a different environment? For example, if the activity is making sandwiches while on a picnic at the beach, it will require that the person utilize his or her knowledge of completing the task in a typical environment (a kitchen) to a beach blanket. Are the objects being used different than typically used or different than what might be used in the client's context? Is only part of the activity being conducted and the client will be expected to apply what is learned to the whole at a later time? Is the activity requiring that a skill be learned that will be applied to different situations?

Awareness of Reality

Distinguishing between thoughts and what is truly occurring requires an awareness of reality. This is how we determine what is real and what is fiction or what we are simply envisioning in our mind. A person who has difficulties with awareness of reality might believe that what he or she sees occur on a television show is actually occurring. Awareness of reality is what allows us to understand what is realistic in our existence (e.g., knowing that we cannot fly if we put a cape around our neck). With this is also an understanding of what is feasible given the context in which the person is and separating what might be envisioned in the mind from what is going on in reality. This requires separating dreams, imagination, delusions, or hallucinations from what is occurring in the true environment.

To determine if this factor is required, think about how much the person is interacting with the environment and others during the activity. Does it require that he or she be able to distinguish between what is real and what is not? Does the activity demand that the person understand what is feasible and realistic given the constraints of the environments (such as making snowballs in the middle of summer)?

Logical/Coherent Thought

For thought processes to be logical and coherent, they are reasonable and can be explained in words or symbols and used for reasoning. Logical reasoning requires using factual information and understanding how it all relates to a problem or situation (Barnard, 1995). Logical thought is what allows our actions to be feasible; we utilize what we know to make decisions that "make sense." Sound reasoning requires this ability to think logically, which is required for many activities that require precise planning and understanding of facts or concepts. This might also be seen as common sense or thinking through a concept using available information. Often, the speed at which an action must be made determines if logical or coherent thought is used. Think about a time you were surprised, caught off-guard, or were in an emergency situation. Did you react logically or in a reactive way? One of my roommates in college ran down three flights of stairs during an earthquake and did not realize what she was doing until she was at the bottom of the stairs and the earthquake was over. This course of action was not logical; if given time to think about it, she might have acted differently. Many of our everyday activities require logical thought, such as balancing a checkbook, grocery shopping, driving, and choosing what clothes to wear.

Appropriate Thought Content

Maintaining a stream of thoughts that relate to the activity or issue is appropriate thought content. When working on writing out a shopping list, we would be thinking about what is needed in regards to food and materials within the home. Thinking about the appropriate things during an activity sounds

---

Activity 5-3

REVIEW OF THOUGHT FUNCTIONS

Identify how each of the following functions is utilized while buying a snack out of a vending machine. Assume that you are already standing in front of the machine, with change in your pants pocket. Leave a row blank if a factor is not used. In the final column, indicate the extent to which each body function is challenged during this activity.

Function	How It Is Used	None	Minimally Challenged	Greatly Challenged
Recognition				
Categorization				
Generalization				
Awareness of reality				
Logical/coherent thought				
Appropriate thought content				

---

much like attention but is different in that this is related to the content of thoughts, not the ability to focus. For example, during a lecture in class, you might be utilizing attention functions to attend to the speaker, but your thought functions to think about the topic being discussed. If the speaker is discussing OT intervention for someone with a cerebrovascular accident and you are thinking about spinal cord injuries, you are not exerting appropriate thought. This is under the category of "thought functions" for a reason; this requires mentally utilizing information that relates to the concept or activity at hand.

When determining if logical thought content is required of an activity, think about what actions are required of the person—does the person need to act in an appropriate way (especially important when interacting with others)? Does the activity require that he or she think about aspects that all relate to the particular topic, such that the ideas or conceptualization utilizes information that is appropriate to the situation? For example, if working on designing a tree house, one must think about the appropriate tools and designs, who will be going into the tree house, and what it will be used for. Going over these concepts is important and appropriate for the task at hand (Activity 5-3). They will not be thinking about other things such as what hair color looks best on Nicole Kidman.

Mental Functions of Sequencing Complex Movement

Execution of Learned Movement Patterns

Executing learned movement patterns, as a cognitive function, is the process of mentally sequencing and coordinating purposeful movements (WHO, 2001). This includes the concept of praxis or motor planning. *Praxis* is the ability to mentally plan and control skilled movements (Zoltan, 2007). When we reach out to pick up a book, it requires not only the strength within our upper extremity but also the mental ability to send the message from our brain to our arm how to move to successfully pick up the book. Without this, our arm might flail about aimlessly or not move at all. This function is not related to physical ability or skill; it is the mental aspect of planning movements. It is separate from understanding what movements are needed, such as thinking about reaching forward to pick up book; it is the mental control over the movements as they are occurring (the execution).

Execution of learned movement patterns is utilized when any purposeful movement is conducted during an activity. So, almost all activities that require physical movement will require sequencing of movement. It is termed *learned movement patterns* in that as we grow and develop as children, we learn

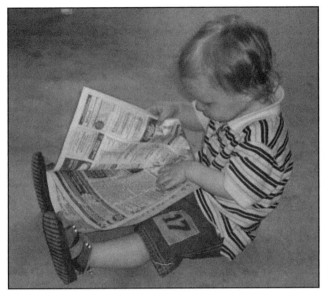

Figure 5-8. Execution of learned movement patterns: turning pages.

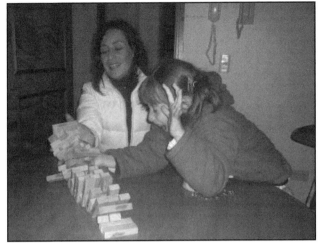

Figure 5-9. Coping and behavioral regulation.

how to control our movements in purposeful ways, as well as how to move in certain situations (see Figure 5-8). For example, the sequencing of movements required for snow skiing is not inherently understood but is learned over time and instruction. Thus, during the activity of skiing, the person engaging in this activity will need to rely on this factor to correctly activate the appropriate muscles and move his or her limbs and trunk in the sequence he or she has learned will allow him or her to safely ski down a hill. So many of our everyday activities require sequencing of motor movements. Think about how much you have done today: showered, got dressed, brushed teeth, styled hair—all of these required sequencing of movements to varying degrees. When determining the extent to which this factor is challenged for an activity, think about how complex the movements are. Are the movements required part of a learned task or activity (much like skiing) and intrinsic to normal development (like picking up a book)?

Emotional

Coping

Coping is related to handling a crisis or decisive turning points in life or situations (WHO, 2001). How actions are carried out or decisions are made during difficult times all involve coping. This is also utilized during times of danger or following a catastrophe. Activities that require coping are those that surround specific contexts or situations. It is often used when a response to a traumatic or negative event is required. For example, a child participating in a spelling bee is going to need coping, as he or she may not win or may be faced with embarrassing failures.

When determining if coping is required of an activity, you must first determine what the most common difficulties or possible dangers are encountered as part of this activity. Take precaution to not fabricate "what if" situations for common activities (such as riding a bike—thinking about what if the person gets hit by a bus). Think of only situations that are most common and likely for that activity. For example, skiing requires very little coping as most of the time the most danger that will require any action would be a large fall. The activity of applying for a new job may take a moderate amount, as rejection from potential employers is a possibility and will require coping to respond positively. Taking a very ill pet that has been part of the family for years to the veterinarian to be euthanized would require a maximal amount of coping.

Behavioral Regulation

As an emotional function, behavioral regulation addresses the affect and display of feelings (WHO, 2001). *Affect* is the physical display of emotions, usually portrayed in facial expressions. For example, when happy, we usually smile. This is a behavior that reflects our emotions. Regulating how we express our emotions is often required for activities that involve other people or when there are social expectations. For example, when playing a game, a child (or an adult for that matter) must learn to control her reactions when she loses, or things do not go as planned (Figure 5-9). This is when it will be important for you to have already examined what the social demands are for the activity that you are analyzing. What are the common social expectations? Of course we can all probably think of an example in which we saw someone demonstrate poor behavioral regulation (think about the fights you have seen or heard about at children's soccer and football games between parents). How many times have you wanted to laugh during a church service or at a time when it was definitely not appropriate to do so? You were utilizing behavioral regulation to downplay your display of emotions during those times.

The amount of behavioral regulation required of an activity is very much based on the social demands of the activity and the chance of error or negative incidents. Is there a chance that the person engaging in the activity will be faced with opposing views, a negative outcome, or errors? Will the person be faced with the possibility of not getting what they had expected or wanted (think of a child in a toy store)? Are there other people involved in this activity that expect certain emotional behavior (for example, the actors involved in the Academy Awards are expected to act happy for their opponents if they do not win an award)?

Experience of Self and Time

Body Image

Body image is related to a person's awareness of the physicality and image of their own body (WHO, 2001). This includes understanding what he or she looks like and his or her own height and weight. This comes into play when choosing clothing or activities to participate in. This is not an awareness of physical ability but having an understanding of one's own body parts and shape. This mental image of what we look like is often disrupted when an amputation or a disfiguring accident occurs.

In determining if this factor is demanded of an activity, think about how the size or shape of the person is important to the activity. Is it important that the person have an accurate understanding of his or her size and shape? Is it important that the person have a concept of what he or she looks like? Does the person need to understand what attributes he or she has and what parts make up his or her entire body? Will his or her understanding of his or her body image shape his or her actions? Perhaps there are social demands of the activity that require an awareness of body image (such as bikini modeling—anyone can wear a bikini, but our society demands a particular body shape for this).

Self-Concept

Having a self-concept is being aware of your roles and identity in the world. This goes beyond understanding how you look, which is addressed in body image; this is addressing who you are and what you understand about your position in the environment (WHO, 2001). Much of what you do every day as an OT student stems from an understanding of who you are as a person and what you believe your role in the world to be. You woke up this morning and made decisions based on this understanding of yourself (like reading this fantastic book). A mother wakes up every day with the understanding that many of the activities she must engage in address her role as a caregiver toward a child.

So, when determining if self-concept is required of an activity, think about whether or not the activity is linked to a social or familial role. Does the activity require that the person understand and know what roles they play in their environment? Does the activity require that the person have a good understanding of who he or she is and how he or she relates to others (for example, understanding gender, age, socioeconomic status)? For example, for a person to attend a support group for women who are divorced, she must first be able to identify herself as having those traits.

Self-Esteem

Self-esteem is a mental function that is demonstrated by confidence in a person's actions and belief in themselves. Actions that exude confidence are assertive and bold and demonstrate assurance in competence (WHO, 2001). Activities that require self-esteem are ones that require the person engaging in them to be able to behave and act in a way that is assertive. The activity may require that the person have confidence in his or her abilities. Having self-esteem is having a belief in oneself. Taking action toward certain activities requires this belief; the person engaging in the activity must believe that he or she has the capability of successfully participating in the task. For example, when you applied to OT school, you had an understanding of yourself as being someone who could be successful as a student in an OT program. This demonstrated a minimal level of self-esteem. You will need to demonstrate a moderate to high level of self-esteem when required to deliver presentations during class or at a conference to people other than your classmates.

To determine if self-esteem is a needed factor for an activity, think about how much interaction with others is required. Does the activity require that the person demonstrate him- or herself in a bold or assertive way? Does the activity ask the person to make decisions based on a belief in him- or herself and his or her abilities? Does the activity present the chance of challenges that require that he or she adhere to a positive belief in him- or herself? For example, in many malls there are small kiosks that hold vendors that sell various items such as sunglasses, hand lotion, or cell phones. The salespeople at these kiosks must have the self confidence to approach strangers, try to convince them to make a purchase, and maintain confidence when rejected or ignored

---

Activity 5-4

REVIEW OF SEQUENCING MOVEMENTS, EMOTIONAL AND EXPERIENCE OF SELF AND TIME FUNCTIONS

Identify how each of the following functions is utilized while buying a snack out of a vending machine. Assume that you are already standing in front of the machine with change in your pants pocket. Leave a row blank if a factor is not used. In the final columns, indicate the extent to which each body function is challenged during this activity.

Function	How It Is Used	None	Minimally Challenged	Greatly Challenged
Execution of learned movements				
Coping				
Behavioral regulation				
Body image				
Self-concept				
Self-esteem				

---

by these strangers. Asking a person out on a date is another example of an activity that requires self-esteem. The person must see him- or herself as a person worth dating and must be assertive enough to invite another person out on a date.

Use Activity 5-4 as a review for this section.

Global Mental Functions

Consciousness

Level of Arousal

Arousal is the ability to demonstrate alertness and respond to stimuli present in the environment (Buckley & Poole, 2004). The quickness to which a person must respond to stimuli and the amount of stimuli presented often determine the level to which arousal is required of an activity. For an activity in which constant diligence and quick reactions are expected, a high level of arousal is required. An example of this might be playing a game of tennis. The person engaged in the game must be on constant alert as to where the ball is going. There are many activities in which we engage every day that demand very little arousal. For example, many people get up in the morning, turn off their alarm clock, take a shower, and get dressed while still half-asleep (low level of arousal).

When determining how much arousal is required of an activity, think about how alert the person must be to things that may occur in the environment. Does the activity require that they react quickly (such as with driving)? Does the activity span over a long period of time where a certain level of arousal must be sustained (sitting through a long lecture)? Does the activity occur at a time when alertness and arousal might be challenged, such as late at night or very early in the morning?

Level of Consciousness

The ICF defines *consciousness* as "the state of awareness and alertness, including the clarity and continuity of the wakeful state" (WHO, 2001, p. 48). Consciousness is often used in medical facilities to describe a person's wakefulness. Consciousness is very much linked to arousal, and in definition sound similar. Consciousness is being awake while arousal level is being able to respond to stimuli in the environment. There are varying levels of each, with people who waver in and out of consciousness (appear to be in and out of sleep), and there are varying levels of alertness from slow to respond to a very heightened state (like someone who has just drank a cup of coffee and is directing a movie). We all function on a daily basis while conscious, so most activities will require this function. However, the level of arousal will vary depending on the demands of the activity (how quickly we need to respond to things in the environment).

Orientation

Orientation to Self

Being oriented to the self includes having an awareness of one's own identity (WHO, 2001). This means the person understands what his or her name is and an idea of who he or she is in relation to others. This is different than self-concept (discussed earlier), which entails understanding who he or she is in society and having a concept of who he or she is as a whole. In most tests for orientation, being oriented to the self entails being able to know your own name (Zoltan, 2007).

Orientation to Place

Orientation to place requires being aware of one's own location. This could include understanding the type of place one currently is in (home, hospital, and hotel) as well as what city, town, or country (WHO, 2001). It is important to note that this is different from topographical orientation, which is the ability to follow a route or navigate through a physical environment to get from one place to another, such as riding a bike from home to a local grocery store (Zoltan, 2007). Orientation to place does not include this type of navigation ability but is simply the understanding of current location. This factor is required of activities that are context specific, meaning that a specific environment is required of the activity in order for it to be successful. For example, one must be in a bathroom and understand that he or she is in a bathroom in order to be successful at the activity of toileting. Another example might be ordering food in a restaurant. It will be essential for the person to understand that he or she is in a restaurant in order to be successful at ordering food.

Orientation to Time

Being aware of the current date, month, day of the week, and year are all part of being oriented to time (WHO, 2001). This also includes having an awareness of approximately what time of day it is. This function is utilized during activities surrounding the environmental conditions, such as an understanding of what time of year it is to determine what clothing to wear. Having an awareness of what year it is also helps shape activities and interactions with others. While working in a nursing home years ago, I met a resident there who was convinced that it was 1962 and that she needed to catch a bus to work. Every morning she would try to get out of the front door of the nursing home, screaming that she was going to miss her bus. She was obviously having difficulties with orientation in time (and also place). Our self-care activities are often shaped by an understanding of what day of the week it is, such as delaying or eliminating certain tasks on weekends when there is not the demand to do so.

Orientation to Others

This mental function includes being aware of the identity of significant people within one's life (WHO, 2001). This includes not only being able to name a significant person in your life but also who he or she is in relation to you. For example, if your mother was to walk in the room, you should be able to identify that the woman is your mother. If a coworker walked up to you, you should be able to identify that he or she is a coworker, not your brother or sister. This is often a challenge for those who suffer from a brain injury or certain types of dementia, in which they mistake a friend for their sister (or even worse—their spouse!). Of course this function relies heavily on memory and perceptual functions (being able to remember names and relationships, and also being able to perceive faces and voices).

Being able to identify others is important in activities that involve others or are oriented toward others. For example, if a person is writing a letter to her old roommate from college, she needs to understand who that person is to her. It would be an unsuccessful activity if she was to write the letter as if writing to her girlfriend from high school. Of course, this factor is of utmost importance when interacting with others. This is demanded during activities that have certain social demands expected of the person engaged in the activity. Perhaps how one behaves toward others is determined by having an understanding of each person's identity.

Orientation to Person

This is listed in the ICF as the category that includes orientation to self and orientation to others which have been previously described (WHO, 2001). Thus, this is not a separate function.

Temperament and Personality

Emotional Stability

Emotional stability is a personality and temperament that is "even-tempered, calm and composed" (WHO, 2001, p. 50). This type of temperament might also be termed *easy-going*. This function allows for interactions and actions that are not laden with irritability or anxiety. The type of temperament or personality a person has is an interesting concept to think about when analyzing the demands of an activity. Does a person need to be easy-going to complete the activity? For the answer to be yes, it most likely will be an activity that entails working with other people, with

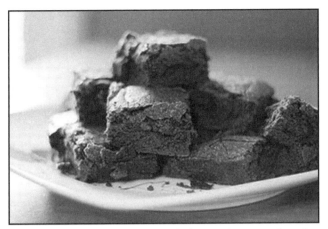

Figure 5-10. Impulse control: brownies may be the ultimate challenge.

difficult issues, or in situations that require a calm environment. For example, in order to lead a relaxation group, the leader would need to demonstrate this function and have a calm demeanor (no high-energy or pressured behavior will help the group relax).

Energy and Drive

Motivation

Motivation is the internal incentive to behave in a certain way or to take action (WHO, 2001). This is what often drives us to participate in activities that are beyond our basic needs. It is what allows us to do more than what is needed just to survive. Our basic self-care needs require minimal motivation to complete. Higher motivation levels are required to complete tasks that have fewer rewards or are greater challenges. For example, if you are reading this book, you are motivated to succeed in your OT program. You needed a certain level of motivation to even apply to OT school. Thus, when determining if motivation is required of an activity, think about what intrinsic or extrinsic rewards there are for engaging in the activity. Basic needs such as breathing and eating require very little motivation, as engaging in the activity itself is motivation (it is necessary to live). However, greater internal motivation is needed to engage in activities that may not be immediately rewarded or may require a great amount of effort (like going to school to earn a degree). If a person is offered a million dollars to run around the block naked, he or she needs less internal motivation, as he or she has an external motivator—the money. However, this person would need to be internally motivated by money in order for this to work. Either way, the person has to be motivated toward one thing or the other—toward the money or the idea of running around the block naked for the sake of doing it.

Impulse Control

Humans learn how to resist internal urges to do or say things from an early age. We learn that there are social demands of many of the things we do every day that do not allow for acting upon spontaneous needs or feelings. For example, we learn as a child that although we may have an intense itch on a private area of our body, we are to resist that impulse to scratch while out in public. This is the impulse control function at work. One must exercise impulse control when on a diet and someone offers freshly baked brownies. The amount of impulse control required of an activity is greatly influenced by the person engaged in the activity. If a person does not like chocolate, passing up a freshly baked brownie may not take much impulse control (see Figure 5-10). However, there are many common traits to humans that allow us to generate estimates of the amount of impulse control required of common activities. For example, maintaining a diet is an activity that typically requires most people a great amount of impulse control. Controlling impulses when around others is something that becomes automatic as we mature and come to understand social expectations. For example, during the activity of eating a meal with others, the impulse to belch out loud must be suppressed. Impulse control might also be exercised during this activity when selecting food and to resist the temptation to take more than a fair share of a certain food item, so that the others eating will have enough to eat.

Appetite

Our natural desire toward things is created by our appetite function. Natural desires are aspects that are physiologically driven (such as food or water) but are also driven by our psychological mechanisms (WHO, 2001). This is what drives us toward satisfying certain needs. This addresses a person's natural desire for certain sensory stimuli, such as the longing for touch. Appetite is often what drives us toward action. It is required of activities such as eating, drinking, smoking, drinking alcohol, sensory stimulating behaviors, and other physiological urges.

Sleep (Physiological Process)

Sleep is a mental function that entails "physical and mental disengagement" from the immediate environment (WHO, 2001, p. 52). Sleep as a physiological process is accompanied by changes in breathing and heart rate patterns, as well as alterations in brain activity. This function is only required of the activities surrounding going to sleep. Thus, dreaming and sleeping are the primary activities in which this factor is required. It is important to note that this factor is not designating the amount of sleep a

---

Activity 5-5

REVIEW OF GLOBAL MENTAL FUNCTIONS

Identify how each of the following functions is utilized while buying a snack out of a vending machine. Assume that you are already standing in front of the machine with change in your pants pocket. Leave a row blank if a factor is not used. In the final columns, indicate the extent to which each body function is challenged during this activity.

Function	How It Is Used	None	Minimally Challenged	Greatly Challenged
Arousal				
Consciousness				
Orientation to self				
Orientation to place				
Orientation to time				
Orientation to others				
Emotional stability				
Motivation				
Impulse control				
Appetite				
Sleep				

---

person achieves and how it affects participation in an activity. For example, it is tempting to state that sleep is required of driving long distances. However, the physiological process of sleeping during the activity of driving would be very dangerous (no sleeping at the wheel). Instead, the level of consciousness and arousal are factors that are in high demand for long-distance driving.

Use Activity 5-5 as a review for this section.

SECTION 2: SENSORY FUNCTIONS AND PAIN

Seeing and Related Functions Including Visual Acuity, Stability, and Visual Field Functions

Detection/Registration

Detecting basic shapes, light, and color of visual stimuli is one of the basic foundations of seeing functions. It is what gives us varying levels of visual acuity, being able to make out and detect various shapes of objects. Detection and registration functions are what allow us to see words on a page, see a dog running across the street, or distinguish the face of a friend (Figure 5-11). Visual detection and registration is required in varying degrees for many daily activities. Activities that require minimal levels of visual detection/registration are many of the basic self-care tasks that utilize larger objects and utilize many of our other senses. For example, when we shower and wash our hair, we are utilizing our sense of touch and proprioception to supplement our vision. We must see enough to get into the shower and where our supplies are.

When determining if visual detection and registration function is needed for an activity, first think about what parts of the activity require that the person see something in the environment on which he or she must act, or what aspects of the activity the person must see while he or she is conducting it. For example, a person must be able to see and detect all in the environment while driving in order to react accordingly using the controls of the car (i.e.,

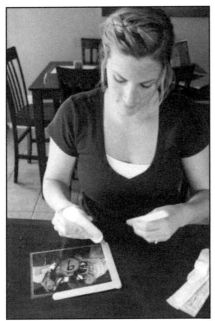

Figure 5-11. Visual detection and registration.

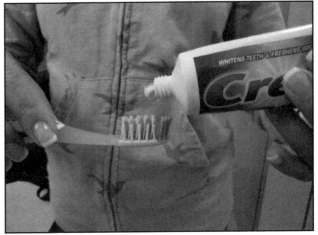

Figure 5-12. Visual modulation.

steering, gas, or brake). There are activities that require detection of the person's actions in order to influence further actions, such as when writing or typing. When handwriting, the person is watching what he or she is writing and where he or she is headed on the page. While typing, the person may watch to see that what he or she hoped to type actually showed up on the page and respond by deleting unwanted characters or continuing on. The amount of challenge that an activity brings to this function depends of the level of acuity required. What amount of detail is needed to be detected? For example, reading the fine print on the packages of many medications or threading a needle requires a high level of visual acuity.

Modulation

Modulating visual stimuli is the ability to regulate and organize the degree and the intensity of the stimuli (Roley & Jacobs, 2009). This is what allows us to limit what we see to keep from being over-stimulated. For example, when putting toothpaste on a toothbrush (Figure 5-12), we are able to organize the visual stimuli so that we are able to filter out nonessential visual information such as what is going on around us or what we might see in the mirror if standing in front of the sink. Modulation of visual stimuli is required of activities that occur in environments where there are other visual stimuli that must be filtered out to allow for visual focus on what is needed for the activity. For example, while driving a car, it is important that the visual information on the dashboard, the stereo, in the passenger seat, and even what is in the rear seat must be modulated so that

those stimuli may be inhibited and the visual stimuli from what is on the road is facilitated. For most of us, we are unaware that we do this on a daily basis in order to be successful in many of our activities. It does not occur to us when we are looking at a computer screen that we are modulating visual information in order to filter out all other stimuli in order to see what we need to see on the screen. Visual modulation may also be needed in situations where the intensity of the visual stimuli may need to be diffused in order to allow for the focus to be on other sensory stimuli. For example, when talking on the phone, we may temper the intensity of visual stimuli in the environment in order to focus on the auditory information.

Integration of Sensations From Body and Environment

Integrating information we receive from other senses from the body and what is occurring in the environment with what we see is what helps us make sense of our actions and what occurs around us. Many actions and activities utilize the collaboration of multiple senses such as sight and touch. Let's go back to the example of picking up a book. You not only use your vision but also your sense of touch and proprioception to feel the edges of the book and pick it up. Integrating what you see with what you feel is what allows you to pick it up correctly and move it.

Integration of senses is required of activities that utilize another sensory system along with vision. Much of this is done subconsciously, so it may take some thought of each step of the activity to determine which senses are being utilized. Many volitional movements toward objects in the environment require this function. Just as with the example of reaching for a book, when interacting with objects we use visual as well as tactile and proprioceptive information to move our bodies to correspond with the object or environment.

Visual Awareness at Various Distances

Visual awareness of the environment includes acuity as well as detection of all within the visual field, which includes objects close to our body as well as those far away. Our visual field includes all that we can see ahead of us as well as on the periphery while still looking ahead (WHO, 2001). Without a full visual field, we would view the world as if looking through a tunnel. What we see in the periphery gives us additional information about the environment and may signal us to action. For example, when walking through a mall while shopping, we walk through crowds and aisles in stores using what we see in our periphery to avoid collision. We also need to be visually aware of not only what is directly in front of us but what is ahead in the distance. This is visual function in action (Figure 5-13).

To determine if visual awareness at various distances is required of an activity, think about the environment in which the activity typically occurs. Where the does the person engaging in the activity need to look? Does he or she need to be aware of the full environment? Does the person need to focus on objects near and far? Does the activity require that the person be aware of all visual stimuli entering the environment? An example would be the activity of playing baseball. The players in the game need to be able to be aware of where the ball and other players are in the environment in all areas of the visual field. Without this, a player may be hit by a ball (or another player).

Hearing Functions

Tolerance of Ambient Sounds

Noise is part of most environments and an element that is a natural part of many activities. For most people, these noises occur without recognition, such as the wind blowing the leaves in the trees or the sound of a toothbrush against our teeth. This factor is what allows us to tolerate these noises and experience them as simply "background noise." The term *ambient* implies those things that are surrounding the natural environment. Thus, when determining if this factor is challenged during the activity that you are analyzing, first think about the environment in which the activity typically occurs. What is usually occurring in the environment that might produce noise? Think about even the smallest noises that perhaps you do not typically notice. For example, the sound of an air conditioner or heater provides a subtle yet constant noise that we must filter out of our awareness. If a great amount of noise occurs in the background of the environment, then a greater level of tolerance of ambient sounds is needed. For example, the activity of skydiving has a great amount of ambient noise,

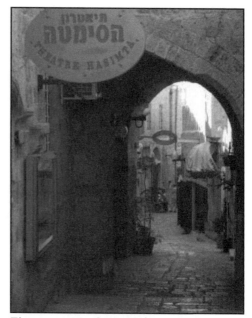

Figure 5-13. Seeing functions: visual awareness at various distances.

from the motor of the airplane and then the sound of air rushing by you as you are plummeting toward the earth at breakneck speed.

Awareness of Location and Distance of Sounds

Part of hearing functions is the ability to be aware of the location and distance of sounds. This is utilized when locating where a sound is coming from and approximately how far away it is. When driving, how do we know an ambulance is headed our way? Our first signal is the sound of the siren. From the sound, we can determine if the ambulance is behind, in front, or to the right or left of us. By the volume level we can determine approximately how far away it is. The same is true of many sounds that we encounter in our daily lives. Think about how you know someone is approaching you from behind or coming down a hallway. As a child, if you ever played hide-and-seek, you utilized this hearing function as you listened for the footsteps and movements of your seeker as you hid (Figure 5-14). You might have even used this function as you took your turn as the seeker, trying to listen for the slightest sound made by those who were hiding. If you heard the floor creak, or a tiny giggle, you would need to use your hearing functions to determine where the sound came from.

While many activities create noise or have sounds that occur during the activity, not all activities demand the use of this hearing function. To determine if this function is required, think about what sounds naturally occur in the environment in which the activity takes place. Are there noises in which the

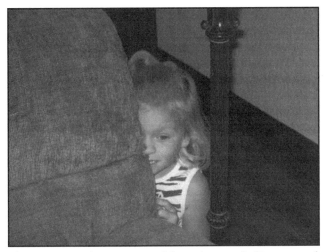

Figure 5-14. Awareness of location and distance of sounds: playing hide-and-seek.

person engaging in the activity must identify from which direction the sound is coming? Do sounds surrounding the person contribute to his or her understanding of what is going on around him or her? An example of this would be walking through a street fair where the noises from different directions tell the person what is occurring around him or her. Also, ask yourself if the sounds he or she hears help determine action, as with the example of the ambulance where the direction and distance of the sound guides the driver toward pulling out of the way of the ambulance as needed.

Vestibular Functions

Sensation of Securely Moving Against Gravity

Our vestibular sense is what allows us to move our bodies in the space around us against the forces of gravity. Without our vestibular sense, we would not be able to move about in our environment. It is what allows us to have a concept of our body position and maintain balance. Our vestibular sense relies on the workings of semicircular canals of the inner ear which sense the position of our head, changes in speed in which our body is traveling, and changes in direction (Dunn, 2009). Having a sense of direction and upright position is foundational to postural control. It is what tells us which way is up or down as we position our body. When you stand up from a seated position, it is your vestibular sense that tells you that you are moving upward and when you have obtained an upright stance. Without this, we might lean to one side or fall over. We might also feel as if we are moving when not. So, in any activity that requires the body to move forward, backward, up, down, or side to side, this factor will be required. It is especially

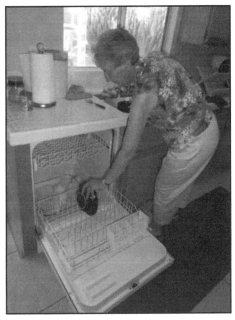

Figure 5-15. Sensation of securely moving against gravity: bending over to load dishwasher.

challenged during activities in which balance is required or if vision is occluded. We use our vision to supplement our vestibular sense in telling us direction and position in space. For example, if you were to bend over to tie your shoes, you watch your surroundings change as you bend forward, giving you information that your position has changed. This, combined with your vestibular and proprioceptive sense, is what allows you to bend forward without falling over and come back up to a standing position when finished. If you were to do this with your eyes closed, you rely only on your vestibular sense to tell you where you are in relation to gravity and your proprioceptive sense to tell you where your limbs and trunk are in relation to each other (Figure 5-15).

When determining if vestibular factors are required of an activity, think about how much the body and head move during the activity. Does the activity require that the person stand and move about? Does the activity require the person to lean forward outside of his or her center of gravity? Does the activity challenge the person's balance, perhaps with limited visual input? Is the body moving forward or side to side, in which the person must determine speed of movement? Does the person's position in space determine further action? An example of this would be if the person was climbing a ladder; the position of the body determines each subsequent movement. Does the position of the head change during the activity, such as leaning the head back to rinse shampoo out in the shower?

Taste Functions

Association of Taste

The ability to taste is a function in which chemicals on the taste buds are broken down into signals representing bitterness, sourness, saltiness, and sweetness (Dunn, 2009; WHO, 2001). While the discrimination of each of these tastes relies on the perceptual abilities of the brain (discussed earlier in this chapter), taste functions are the abilities of the tongue to detect chemicals and send neural signals regarding each of the chemicals presented. Taste functions come into play with activities surrounding eating or drinking or any activity in which there will be contact with the tongue. This function is highly challenged in those who must determine differences in ingredients or the level of sweetness or bitterness in foods, such as in a chef or wine critic. For most of us, some level of taste functions is required to motivate us to eat or drink and to determine if an item we are ingesting is safe to eat. This relies on the brain's ability to perceive the signals sent regarding these different foods.

Smell Functions

Association of Smell

Sense of smell is the ability to sense odors and smells in the environment (WHO, 2001). Our sense of smell requires our nose to receive chemicals in the air and send signals regarding these chemicals to the brain. It is here that smell is perceived and the type of smell is distinguished (see perceptual functions discussed earlier in this chapter). Smells can be associated to objects, environments, people, or situations. Our sense of smell has been linked to our memory and emotions (Dunn, 2009). Smells can alert us of situations that require action, such as a bad body odor or the smell of smoke. Odors can also be soothing and comforting or alerting and cause discomfort. The sense of smell is required of activities that give us information regarding the environment. We need to be able to detect changes in the environment or if something requires action (e.g., the dog relieved himself in the corner).

Proprioception Functions

Awareness of Body Position and Space

Our ability to determine where our body parts are moving and in which direction they are moving or are being held in is controlled by sensory receptors in our muscles, tendons, and joints (Dunn, 2009). Muscle spindles are the sensory component that detect muscle length, telling us how much a muscle is stretched or contracted. Golgi tendon organs receive

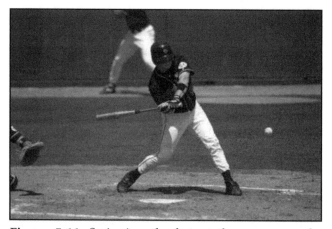

Figure 5-16. Swinging the bat at the proper angle challenges the awareness of body position and space.

information about joint movement by detecting movement of tendons that surround the joints of our body. These two sensory receptors send information creating an awareness of where each of our body parts are in relation to each other and in space (WHO, 2001). To understand what these signals mean, this sense also requires the perceptual abilities of the brain to interpret the information sent from the proprioceptive receptors in the body.

All activities that require movement utilize at least a small degree of proprioceptive sense. Activities that occur outside of the range of sight require a higher level of this factor, as the person must rely on his or her ability to sense where his or her body part is instead of seeing it. An example of this is when playing baseball or softball (Figure 5-16). When standing holding a bat, the bat is held up and behind the head. It is the proprioceptive functions that give information regarding the position of our body and how we are positioning the bat.

Touch Functions

Comfort With the Feeling of Being Touched

Our ability to tolerate and utilize the sensation of touch is employed throughout many of our daily activities, much of which occurs without our awareness. As you sit reading this book, are you aware of how your clothing is touching your skin? Or how the book is touching the skin of your hands? Probably not, because your touch functions are at work, allowing you to be comfortable with objects and different textures touching your skin. Any time we come in contact with an object or something is placed against us or in our mouth, we are drawing upon our ability to be comfortable and regulate the sensation. Without this, we would have difficulty wearing

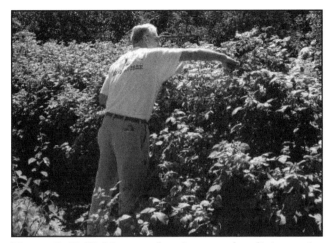

Figure 5-17. Picking raspberries uses localizing pain to feel thorns.

clothes, washing ourselves, and even brushing our hair. Objects and materials that come in contact with our bodies come in a variety of consistencies and textures. For example, the texture of sandpaper is one that, for most people, is not a sensation that is comfortable against the skin. Many people feel the same about softer, slippery substances such as slugs.

If the activity you are analyzing requires contact with others (such as a hug, holding hands, or even bumping into each other in passing) or contact with objects, this factor is utilized. Also, think about what type of clothing or equipment must be worn on the body. To scuba dive in cold water, one must be comfortable with a wet suit covering and pressing against the body. There is also a face mask that presses against the skin and sand against the feet and between the toes. Comfort with touch also comes into play when eating various consistencies of food. For example, many people have difficulty eating oysters due to the slimy and chewy consistency. Thus, it will be important to think about the consistency of the foods in the case of analyzing the activity of eating. Because we utilize our hands for so much of what we do, think also about what the hands come in contact with during the activity.

Pain

Localizing Pain

Being able to identify when potential or actual damage may be occurring to a part of the body and where it is occurring is essential to maintaining our own safety. Localizing where the pain is coming from requires the functioning of pain receptors in the body part that is being inflicted with an insult. These signals allow us to quickly know which part of the body is in danger and react, such as pulling

away or caring for the injury. It is pain that alerts us that something is wrong and signals toward action. For example, as Richard is out gardening and picking raspberries, he feels a sharp pain in one of his fingers (Figure 5-17). Upon inspection, he finds that a small splinter has lodged itself under the skin in his finger. The area continues to hurt, so he promptly pulls the splinter out and washes the area. Without the signal that the splinter was there, the area would have become infected, and he could have eventually lost the finger to amputation, all from a simple splinter. It is discomfort that signals us to change position and even to shift in our seat when sitting for periods of time. Without this feeling of discomfort, we might sit for hours in one position, putting us at risk for sores on the backside. Notice how many times you shift in your seat as you continue to read on.

Activities that utilize this function are ones in which action is required in response to discomfort and being able to determine where on the body the pain is coming from. The pain might be a limiter, signaling the person to stop a particular action or keep the person safe during the activity. An example of this would be lifting a heavy object. Does the activity present the chance of injury? Does the environment in which the activity commonly occurs have elements that could cause harm? For example, hiking in the woods occurs in areas in which branches and plants can cause scratches and animals can bite.

Temperature and Pressure

Thermal Awareness

Another sensation function that alerts to possible harm is *thermal awareness*, which is the ability to sense heat and cold (WHO, 2001) (Figure 5-18). We may use a part of our body to feel if an object is hot or cold, such as feeling bath water before stepping into it or placing gloves over our hands when sensing that it is too cold out. These sensations guide our actions and choices in tasks (to place gloves on or not). We use this sensory function when eating as well (determining if what we are eating is hot or cold).

To determine if this function is demanded of an activity, think about what objects and materials are involved in the activity. Does the person interact with or touch those objects? What is the typical environment of the activity? For example, if walking across the beach, it will be important to know how hot the sand it before walking across it barefoot. Thus, think about the effect the environment might have on the person's body or on objects.

Use Activity 5-6 as a review for this section.

Activity 5-6

REVIEW OF SENSORY FUNCTIONS AND PAIN

Identify how each of the following functions is utilized while buying a snack out of a vending machine. Assume that you are already standing in front of the machine with change in your pants pocket. Leave a row blank if a factor is not used. In the final columns, indicate the extent to which each of the body functions is challenged during this activity.

Function	*How It Is Used*	*None*	*Minimally Challenged*	*Greatly Challenged*
Detection/ registration				
Visual modulation				
Integration of senses				
Awareness at distances				
Tolerance of ambient sounds				
Location and distance of sounds				
Moving against gravity				
Taste				
Smell				
Body and space				
Comfort with touch				
Localizing pain				
Thermal awareness				

SECTION 3:
NEUROMUSCULOSKELETAL AND MOVEMENT–RELATED FUNCTIONS

Functions of Joints and Bones

Joint Mobility

The ease in which a joint moves through motion is termed *range of motion* (WHO, 2001). The degree to which range of motion is required of an activity requires careful analysis of all of the movements that typically occur during the activity. It is important to consider the demands on all of the joints in the body: fingers, spine, hips, knees, ankles, just to name a few. An understanding of what comprises full range capabilities of each joints will enable you to determine the extent to which each joint is challenged. For example, using the facts about normal range of

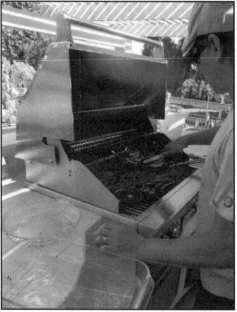

Figure 5-18. Barbecueing challenges thermal awareness.

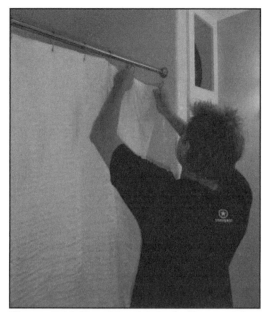

Figure 5-19. Reaching high challenges joint mobility.

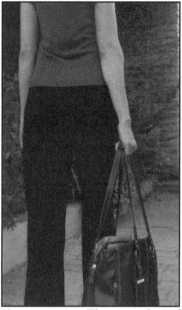

Figure 5-20. The weight of carrying a heavy bag pulls on joints, challenging joint stability.

motion that maximal flexion is approximately 180 degrees, when analyzing the activity of placing cups in a cupboard that is eye level we find that this activity only moderately challenges shoulder flexion. Hanging a shower curtain would provide a maximal challenge for shoulder flexion (for a person of average height) (Figure 5-19). Be sure to consider both ends of range (both flexion and extension), as some activities require greater extension than flexion, such as playing tennis, which requires full elbow extension.

Caution should also be made to not confuse range of motion with strength. Neither the weight of the objects used nor the number of repetitions is of importance here. Range of motion is not a consideration of muscle strength but of the ability of the joint to move smoothly. To determine the extent to which this factor is utilized, identify which body parts move and which are attached to the joints that allow them to move. To what extent is each joint moved through potential range of motion? Is the body part moved minimally and thus through smaller degrees of movement, or does the body part move toward the end ranges of flexion or extension?

Joint Stability

Joint Postural Alignment

The stability of a joint is what allows for proper alignment of the joint. Stability is a function of structural integrity of the joints (WHO, 2001). It is the structure and stability of joints that keeps bones in proper alignment with each other allowing for functional use of the body parts and trunk. Without

this, our limbs might land outside of alignment, or put extra strain on other parts. An example of when joint postural alignment goes awry is shoulder dislocations or scoliosis of the spine.

The alignment of joints is challenged in activities that stress the stability of a joint. Having proper joint alignment will be important in activities if a joint is to be moved through more than minimal range of motion. It is also needed if stress will be placed on the joint, such as carrying a heavy bag in the hand, causing stress on the joints of the fingers as well as shoulder (Figure 5-20).

Muscle Power

Strength

The force in which a body part must move or hold an object requires the functions of muscle power. An activity may require the power of one muscle, a group of muscles, or muscles throughout the body or trunk. This includes maintaining postures such as the muscle contractions required to stand upright. Muscle power requirements vary according to the environmental challenges and the exertion made against gravity. For example, walking up a steep hill requires a greater amount of strength versus walking on a flat surface. The amount of muscle strength required will be much less if using gravity as an assist, such as reaching down to the ground, versus moving against the forces of gravity, such as standing up from the floor. The muscle challenge may come from moving the weight of an object or body weight such as used in doing a push-up.

There are times when detailed analysis of exactly which muscles are used during an activity is required. This has been termed *muscular analysis* and is utilized by other disciplines such as physical therapy (Bukowski, 2000). Being able to dissect the movements required into the exact muscles utilized during an activity requires knowledge of kinesiology principles. It is beyond the scope of this book to go into detail regarding anatomy and kinesiology. It is important however to be able to identify the major muscle movements. It is through muscular analysis that clinicians often find that "just right challenge" for their clients. If working with a client who needs to strengthen his or her wrist supinators, how would you decide on an activity that would work on this? Clinicians often must mentally analyze the muscular demands of several activities to find one that meets the need. Muscular analysis is also helpful in gaining awareness of what activities your client might have difficulties with, given a certain muscle power deficit (Figure 5-21). For example, if you have a client who has weakness in elbow flexion, you can begin to think about what basic self-care skills require elbow flexion that your client might have difficulties with (self-feeding, brushing teeth, pulling up pants).

It is important to recognize each of the movements required and the demand on the muscles not only for the upper extremities but for the trunk, hips, and entire lower extremities as well. Refer back to the steps you determined were needed to complete the activity. In steps where the body is used to support or move an object, or the body must hold itself up against gravity, you must determine what type of muscle action occurred— isometric, isotonic, or eccentric contractions. Isometric contractions occur when there is no actual movement but muscles are contracting in order to hold a body part or joint in place (Breines, 2009). You utilize isometric contractions while holding this book. To hold the book still, you are utilizing the muscles in your hands and perhaps other muscles in your upper extremities, depending on if you have the book set on a surface or not. You utilize isometric contractions of these muscles to hold the book in a static position. If you were to lift up the book, you would be creating an isotonic contraction. This is when muscles actually shorten during the contraction (Breines, 2009). Even without lifting an object, any movement that requires the muscle to shorten would be considered an isotonic contraction. Eccentric contraction occurs when releasing this tension and elongating the muscle. For example, if setting this book down on the ground, one would contract the biceps and then slowly allow it to release

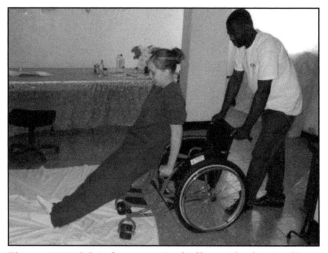

Figure 5-21. Muscle power is challenged when a client must lift herself from the floor into a wheelchair.

as to slowly lower the book to the floor. Because gravity is assisting in pulling the book toward the floor, the biceps are still contracting to hold it up but are slowly releasing the contraction to allow the arm to straighten. You would not be using the triceps to extend the arm unless you were forcefully throwing the book to the floor (which I do not recommend). Determining which type of contraction occurs will help in determining the extent to which muscle power is required of the activity you are analyzing (Activity 5-7).

Muscle Tone

Muscle tone is the natural tension that is present in muscles when at rest. This tension is what creates resistance or the lack of resistance when a body part is moved passively (WHO, 2001). Normal tone is required to allow for smooth muscle control (Preston, 2009). In order for muscles to work together to move a body part, one must work as the agonist muscle and contract, while the opposite muscle, the antagonist, must allow for passive movement. For example, when bringing a spoon to your mouth, your biceps shorten, while the triceps elongate. If the triceps had abnormally high tone, the biceps would find it more difficult to flex the elbow smoothly.

The *Framework* lists several types of abnormal muscle tone, such as when tone is absent (flaccidity), high (hypertonic), increases when presented with quick passive stretch (spasticity), or fluctuating between high and low tone (AOTA, 2008; Preston, 2009). Because abnormal tone would be a hindrance to performance in activities, these types of tone are not demanded of activities. Instead, we will analyze the need for normal tone during an activity. Normal tone is necessary for activities in which a muscle will

Activity 5-7

MUSCULAR ANALYSIS

Complete a muscular analysis of getting a snack out of a vending machine.

Muscle	Not Used	Minimally Challenged	Greatly Challenged
Shoulder flexion			
Shoulder extension			
Shoulder abduction			
Shoulder adduction			
Shoulder internal rotation			
Shoulder external rotation			
Elbow flexion			
Elbow extension			
Wrist supination			
Wrist pronation			
Wrist flexion			
Wrist extension			
Thumb flexion			
Thumb abduction			
Finger flexion			
Finger extension			
Trunk flexion			
Trunk extension			
Trunk rotation			
Lower extremities			

be passively stretched. For example, if reaching down to your feet to tie your shoes, the muscles in your back must have a normal level of tone to provide some resistance but not so high in resistance to prevent you from flexing your trunk forward. Normal tone is also a prerequisite for smooth movements. Think about when you go to take a drink out of a cup. You pick it up and slowly bring it to your mouth. If your tone is normal, the triceps elongates nicely and your biceps continues on its course in curling the cup toward your mouth. However, if your triceps was hypertonic or had fluctuating tone, it might cause the muscle to contract, extending the arm, and then the biceps would try to continue in its course by flexing the arm, and now you have your drink all over your lap. So, think about how essential smooth movements are to the activity you are analyzing.

Muscle Endurance

Endurance

Muscle endurance is required when the contraction of a muscle must be maintained for a prolonged period of time (WHO, 2001). Activities such as standing for long periods or holding an extremity in a static, isometric contraction such as carrying a box both require muscle endurance. The longer the muscle is required to maintain a contraction, the more this is in demand. Muscle endurance could also be required when repetitive muscle contractions occur over a long period of time with minimal or no rest breaks (Figure 5-22). For example, painting a house requires the endurance of upper extremity muscles to repeat the same motions over and over again.

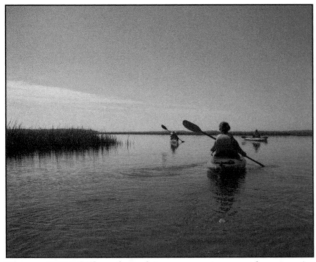

Figure 5-22. When kayaking up a river, endurance is challenged in order to continue paddling to get back.

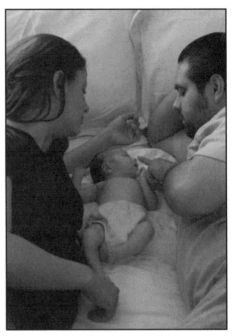

Figure 5-23. These are examples of asymmetrical tonic neck reflex.

To determine the extent to which muscles are challenged to sustain contraction, take a look at the steps required of the activity—how long do some of the steps last? Do some of these steps require continuous action of the same muscle groups? Does the person stand or use trunk muscles throughout? Are there rest breaks during the activity? This would reduce the demand for muscle endurance. If there is a multitude of muscles used during the activity and there are not certain muscles or muscle groups that must sustain a contraction, this function is not required or is minimally challenged.

Motor Reflexes

Stretch Reflex

Functions of involuntary contractions of muscles are automatically induced by stretching.

Reflexes are motor movements and responses to sensory stimuli. A stretch reflex occurs when a muscle is stretched to the point in which an involuntary contraction of the muscle is induced (WHO, 2001). This is a protective response of the muscle to prevent overstretching. This is controlled by receptors in the muscles, called *muscle spindles*, which send signals to the spinal cord regarding length of the muscle (Preston, 2009). This occurs without the person's intent or involvement. The stretch reflex is utilized during activities in which muscles are stretched to end ranges. Our stretch reflexes prohibit stretching the muscles too far. Yoga is an example of when this protective reflex is utilized, during movements requiring deep stretches. This function will only be utilized if there is a chance of muscles being stretched to great lengths. For many sporting activities, this reflex prevents many injuries.

Asymmetrical Tonic Neck Reflex

Asymmetrical tonic neck reflex (ATNR) is a primitive reflex that is present in infants and disappears by three to four months of age. This reflex serves a good purpose in those first few months of life, in that it prevents an infant from rolling over before it is motorically and neurologically ready (*Mosby's Dictionary*, 2006). When the head is turned to one side, the extensor tone on the side in which the person is facing increases, and the flexor tone on the opposite side increases (Preston, 2009). So, if an infant turns its head to the right, the right arm will extend and the left will flex (Figure 5-23). The occurrence of this reflex in an adult is not normal and can interfere with functional movements. Thus, ATNR will not be needed for activities of an adult and will only be utilized as a protective reaction in infants up to 4 months.

Symmetrical Tonic Neck Reflex

Symmetrical tonic neck reflex (STNR) is also a primitive reflex that is helpful only in infants and recedes after the first year of life. STNR causes two different actions with head flexion and extension. With head flexion, the upper extremities go into flexion and the lower extremities go into extension. When the head is extended, the upper extremities go into extension and the lower extremities go into flexion (Preston, 2009). This is often called the *crawling reflex*, which allows infants to get into the crawling position (*Mosby's Dictionary*, 2006). This reflex does

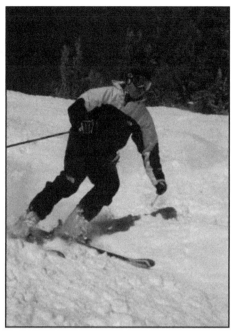

Figure 5-24. Righting and supporting can be challenged when the environment changes the position of the body.

not allow for actual crawling, but allows them to get into the quadruped position. This factor will only be functional for infants in the first year of life.

Involuntary Movement Reactions

Righting and Supporting

Our bodies have natural reactions that are designed to protect us and allow us to restore our bodies to a natural upright position. When we sense our balance is threatened, or that we might be falling, our bodies automatically react to restore alignment of the trunk by increasing tone in the trunk or limbs (WHO, 2001). These automatic reactions to being thrown off balance are often what keep up from falling. We do this by moving our feet or legs, extending our arms to help to regain balance, and shift our head in a direction that will assist in regaining balance.

This function is especially important during activities where there is a chance of the position of the body being suddenly shifted. If the body is thrown or shifted from an upright position by another person, object, or the environment, the person will utilize his or her righting reactions to keep from falling and to regain an upright position. An example of how the environment can often challenge this factor during an activity is during snow skiing (Figure 5-24). As skis go over the different terrain, the body is shifted into different directions and often thrown outside of the center of gravity. The skier's body

automatically contracts muscles to help maintain an upright position. Without this, with every little bump that the skier goes over, he or she would find him- or herself tumbling down the hill. Righting reactions are also utilized any time the body is moved from the upright position, such as when getting up from the ground (much like the skier would have to do if he or she tumbled down the hill) or when coming up from a supine position such is lying in bed.

This function is required if sudden, unexpected events cause the person to be thrown off balance or shifted from an upright position. Think about the environment in which the activity occurs—are there obstacles or other people that could arise and cause a shift in balance? Does the activity require that the person reach outside of the center of gravity or bend downward and then regain an upright position? Think about the various positions that the person will be in during the activity and if the person must regain an upright position.

Control of Voluntary Movement

Eye–Hand/Foot Coordination

Moving in simple and complex ways requires coordinating many different body functions. Eye–hand (or foot) coordination requires utilizing what is visually perceived in the environment to contract and control muscle groups to move in a coordinated fashion. For example, when we reach for our toothbrush, we are using visual information to control how and where we reach. When placing toothpaste on the toothbrush, we again are coordinating what we do with our hands with what we see to assure that the toothpaste ends up on the toothbrush and not in the sink.

We utilize this connection between visual stimuli and movement in all activities where there is visual information that guides our movements. Handwriting is an example of using eye–hand coordination. We use it in many everyday self-care activities, such as grabbing toilet paper, scooping up food in a spoon, and washing our hands. The level of challenge to this factor comes with the demand for precision of movements and timing. For example, catching a quickly moving ball requires a high level of eye–hand coordination due to the timing of coordinating movements with the visual stimuli of the moving ball. Eye–foot coordination functions in the same way, coordinating what is visually seen with what the lower extremities are doing, such as when kicking a ball (Figure 5-25) or pushing the brake on a car in response to a small child running across the street. The demand for precise movements is another reason there might be a high level of eye–hand coordination needed. For example, threading a needle requires very

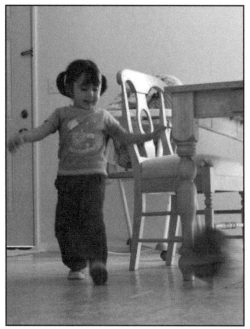

Figure 5-25. Eye-foot coordination is used in kicking a ball.

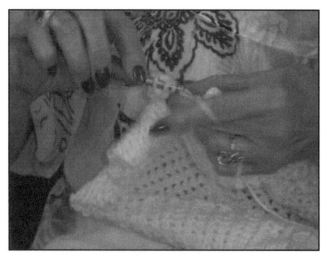

Figure 5-26. Bilateral coordination is used in knitting.

precise hand movements using the visual stimuli of the direction of the thread as it aims toward the small hole of the needle. In determining if this factor is utilized or not, think about how much the person must visually attend to an object or environment in order to guide movements. If the steps can be done out of sight, or without visual information, eye–hand coordination is not essential to the task.

Bilateral Integration

Bilateral integration occurs when both arms or both legs are used collaboratively to complete a task. One extremity can work in conjunction with the other actively or as an assist. When both extremities are actively involved in the activity, each hand, arm, or leg has its own actions that work in collaboration with the other. An example of this is opening a jar or bottle. One hand grasps the bottle, while the other twists off the lid. If passively collaborating, a limb may be used to stabilize an object while the other one is active. An example of this is writing. The nondominant hand holds the piece of paper down, while the other hand does the writing. In the case where the bilateral coordination consists of one extremity being a stabilizer, the level of challenge is low, as there is little to no movement required of one extremity. Higher level challenges occur when each hand and its fingers have individual movements. An example of this is when tying shoelaces or knitting (Figure 5-26).

To begin to understand if this factor is used in an activity, begin by thinking about what objects are manipulated or moved with either the arms or the legs. Does it take the use of both sides? Do the hands have to work together to complete steps of the activity? Perhaps the lower extremities must work together to manipulate an object. Does an object need to be stabilized while the other extremity does more of the action toward the object? Is each hand performing separate movements (indicating higher demand)?

Crossing Midline

The *midline* is the imaginary line that runs through the center of the body dividing it into right and left halves (*Mosby's Dictionary*, 2006). Crossing midline occurs when right side of the body crosses over into the left side's territory or vice versa. When a person uses his or her right hand to brush the left side of his or her head, he or she crosses midline. If we reach with our right hand to pick up a cup that is on our left side, we are crossing midline. Any time our extremities or trunk cross over into the opposite side, the muscles of our trunk must collaborate with the movement of our extremities. Using the example of reaching to the left to grab a cup, our trunk muscles must contract and turn the trunk to the left to allow the hand to reach the cup. Crossing midline may not require the trunk to twist or even move, but it may require the trunk to contract muscles in order to stabilize and keep the body from tipping over. This all occurs without our awareness but allows us to dynamically interact with the surrounding environment. Without this, we would only conduct tasks within reach, in a static position not reaching across our body or leaning to either side.

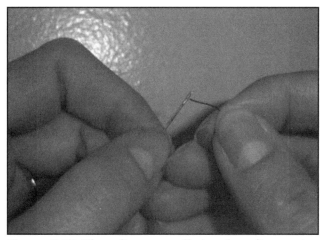

Figure 5-27. Threading a needle involves fine motor coordination.

Activities that require crossing midline are activities that require dynamic movement of the trunk and movements of the extremities toward the opposite side of origin. Imagine a line down the center of the body. During the activity, does the right side ever come over into the left, or the left into the right? This includes areas of the trunk that shift from midline. Does the activity require reaching? Does the activity require the legs to cross over one another? Think about the direction of the head—does it cross over into one side or the other?

Fine Motor Control

Fine motor movements are those that utilize the smaller muscles of the hand, fingers, and thumb. These muscles allow for precise movements used to manipulate smaller objects. This includes picking up and releasing small objects, grasping objects with the hand (such as a door knob), and pinching between the thumb and fingers. The extent to which fine motor is utilized during an activity is greatly influenced by the size and shape of objects used in the activity. For example, in the activity of dressing there is greater challenge if dressing formally in a dress shirt with small buttons and pants with a zipper, versus the little fine motor needed to don a T-shirt and sweatpants. Fine motor will still be utilized to put on these simpler clothing items when pinching and grasping the material to pull it on the body.

Most fine motor movements require the use of the hands. Fine motor will be required of any activity that requires the hand to grasp and release an object. The grasp may require all of the fingers to work together with the thumb, such as picking up a ball, or use individual fingers such as holding a key. The extent to which fine motor is challenged is determined by the size and shape of the objects used and the demand for

precision in the movements. To again use the example of threading a needle, very precise movements are required to move the thread into a very small hole (Figure 5-27). Fine motor movements do not just occur when there is an object to grasp but also occur when individual finger movements are required such as when playing a musical instrument like the piano or guitar. Individual finger and thumb movements are also required in typing on a keyboard and using a cell phone. Without these precise movements, we might be sending strange text messages to the wrong people.

Gross Motor Control

Gross motor control is when the larger muscles of the body are used to coordinate movements. Actions such as throwing, jumping, or kicking are all examples of gross motor movements. Gross motor movements are also considered larger movements, without the demand for small and precise control of actions. These larger movements typically use the larger muscles of the body, such as the quadriceps, biceps, triceps, deltoids, and pectoral muscles (this is just a few of the many possible). Gross motor movements can also utilize smaller muscles when utilized in combination with each other. An example of this is when the finger flexors of the hand are contracted together to create a "gross grasp" where there is no specific prehension pattern created, because there is no isolated contraction of one of the smaller muscles of the hand. Movements of the trunk are also considered gross motor movements, as they are utilizing larger muscles and typically produce larger, less precise movements. The speed in which the limb or trunk is moved is also part of gross motor control. We utilize gross motor control throughout our daily activities. It is what allows us to bring food to our mouths without spilling it across our lap. We use it to guide our limbs into clothing and to move our arms in a direction to give us an acceptable hair style. Without gross motor control, we might spend a bit of time hitting ourselves or making a mess while doing these activities. If you were to try brushing or combing your hair with jerky arm movements, you probably would end up with a very wild hair style.

To determine if gross motor control is utilized during an activity, think about the movements made during the activity. Are they broad and large or small and precise? Think about what joints are moving—are the joints controlled by larger muscles like the shoulder, hips, knees, or elbows? How much does the trunk move? How much do the gross motor movements need to be coordinated and have few extraneous movements? There are some activities that are very forgiving in the amount of coordination needed, where other activities require a greater level

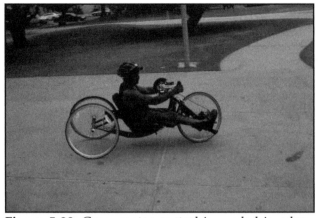

Figure 5-28. Gross motor control is needed in adaptive bicycling.

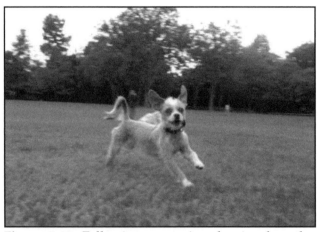

Figure 5-29. Following a running dog involves the oculomotor control of pursuits.

of accuracy in movements (Figure 5-28). For example, washing a car utilizes large movements of the arms to move the sponge across the surface of the car, without need for exact coordination of movements. However, when picking up a glass and placing it in a cupboard, greater accuracy of movement is required or the glass will hit the cupboard or another glass and shatter. Think about how quickly the limb or trunk must move and then slow down—does this regulation of speed influence success? For example, if swinging a bat to hit a baseball, one must coordinate a quick contraction of the arms and trunk but then conclude the contraction very quickly. This is also part of gross motor control—being able to start and stop contractions at the appropriate time, as well as control the speed in which the limb is moving. How much would extraneous movements interfere with success in this activity?

Oculomotor Control

Motor control of the eye muscles allows for detection of visual information in the environment and requires multiple types of coordination. *Saccades* are rapid eye movements from one aspect in the environment to the other, without movement of the head or body (Zoltan, 2007). Moving our eyes from one point to another smoothly allows us to gather information about the world around us. For example, as you read this sentence, your eyes are moving smoothly across the page and seeing each word. When your eyes reach the end of a line, they swiftly and smoothly shift to the left and down to the next line. Reading is a perfect example of when saccadic eye movements are required.

Another type of oculomotor control is *pursuits*. This is where the eyes follow a moving object and keep it in focus (Zoltan, 2007). For example, to look at a bird flying in the sky, the muscles in your eyes must work to move along with the bird to keep it in your sight. Thus, the term *pursuits* is fitting, as the eyes

are pursuing or chasing a moving object. Examples of activities that utilize this are watching or playing baseball, playing with a dog (Figure 5-29), or playing a video game.

Accommodation occurs when the eye muscles must coordinate to allow for looking at objects near and far, or when an object is changing distance from near to far (or vice versa) (Zoltan, 2007). Our eyes accommodate to changing the distance; they must focus when we take notes in class in front of us and then look up at the instructor in front of the class. Our eyes must refocus at a different distance. This also occurs when we are visually attending to an object that is traveling toward or away from us. An example of when this occurs continuously is when driving. We visually see cars approach us as well as move away.

Oculomotor control has the challenging task of binocularity, where it must coordinate the movement of two eyes in exactly the same way in order to maintain view of an object. That means that if watching a car that is traveling left to right, both eyes must be fixated and following the car at the same rate. Without coordination of both of the eyes, we see double (which is called *diplopia*) (Warren, 2009). Paralysis or changes in muscle tone of one eye can cause difficulty in ability to move both eyes in the same manner. The ability to coordinate the eyes together is what allows us to accurately determine where an object is in space. It provides us with information as to distance and placement of objects. For example, when we reach for a cup sitting on a table, both of our eyes focus on it and we reach forward based on the visual information we receive on where it is—to the left or right and how far forward. A person with double vision or the lack of binocularity might see two cups and have a misperception of how far away the cup is. They might grasp too close or too far away and knock the cup over.

Activity 5-8

REVIEW OF NEUROMUSCULOSKELETAL AND MOVEMENT-RELATED FUNCTIONS

Identify how each of the following functions is utilized while buying a snack out of a vending machine. Assume that you are already standing in front of the machine with change in your pants pocket. Leave a row blank if a factor is not used. In the final columns, indicate the extent to which each body function is challenged during this activity.

Function	How It Is Used	None	Minimally Challenged	Greatly Challenged
Joint range of motion				
Joint stability/alignment				
Strength				
Muscle tone				
Muscle endurance				
Stretch reflex				
ATNR				
STNR				
Righting and supporting reflex				
Eye–hand coordination				
Eye–foot coordination				
Bilateral coordination				
Crossing midline				
Fine motor control				
Gross motor control				
Oculomotor control				
Gait patterns				

To determine if oculomotor control is utilized during an activity, think about how much visual tracking and focus is required. Does the activity require that the person look at objects, either stationary or moving? Does it require that the person look across the environment, moving the eyes in a swift but coordinated manner (e.g., when reading)? Is the perception of depth or position important (as used with binocularity)? Think about what objects are used or are part of the environment—are the eyes required to move in order to see these objects? Does the person need to look near to far or see objects as they move closer to them? To what extent do smooth movements of the eyes influence success in this activity? How much is coordination of the eyes challenged during the activity to move smoothly at the appropriate rate?

Gait Patterns

Gait patterns are related to the movements used to walk. These patterns are important to OT practitioners in how they relate to the ability to engage in occupations. Thus, walking in a grocery store or during the preparation of a meal is within our domain, while the simple action of walking without engagement in an occupation is not. A normal gait pattern includes the use of both legs interchangeably, shifting body weight from one leg to the other (Bolding, Adler, Tipton-Bruton, & Lillie, 2009). This requires coordination of each leg to swing forward as the other leg maintains balance. The cadence or rate in which all of this occurs is also a component of normal gait patterns.

In analyzing the demand for gait patterns in an activity, the first step is to determine if any walking is required and, if so, how much. How important is it that the person have a "normal" gait pattern? The purpose of the walking as well as the social demands surrounding the activity may be what determines the extent to which a normal gait pattern is required. For example, a person who decides to do runway modeling will definitely need to walk and walk with a certain gait pattern. Distance and terrain of the environment may also challenge the need for gait patterns. If hiking a mountain, a higher level of gait patterns is required versus those needed to walk in a grocery store.

Use Activity 5-8 as a review for this section.

SECTION 4: FUNCTIONS OF CARDIOVASCULAR, HEMATOLOGICAL, IMMUNOLOGICAL, AND RESPIRATORY SYSTEMS

Cardiovascular System Function

Blood Pressure Functions

Blood pressure is the amount of pressure that is exerted by the blood on the walls of the veins and arteries of the body. This pressure is regulated by the amount in which the heart muscles contract, the volume of blood in certain areas of the body, and contraction or dilation of the arteries (*Mosby's Dictionary*, 2006). For example, when sitting for a long period of time, more blood tends to pool in the legs. When we stand suddenly, our body must work hard to maintain proper blood pressure throughout the body or we might feel dizzy from a lack of blood pressure in the brain (this is called *orthostatic hypotension—* decreased blood pressure when changing position). Our blood pressure normally rises with activity as our heart pumps harder and faster. Blood pressure can be challenged by physical challenges as well as psychological ones. For example, heart rate and blood pressure may be challenged when digging in the garden, as well as when giving a speech in front of a large audience (Figure 5-30). The psychological response to stressful situations is controlled by the autonomic nervous system which controls heart rate, blood pressure, and other body functions when confronted with positive or negative stress (White, 2009).

Blood pressure is a normal function of staying alive, but how much it is challenged during an activity is based on many factors. Activities in which the position of the body is changed rapidly will challenge the body's ability to maintain normal blood pressure. If you have ever been on a roller coaster that drops suddenly, you may have felt slightly light-headed as your body tried to regain normal blood pressure in your brain. Activities that may stimulate the autonomic nervous system will challenge blood pressure, as the body reacts to stressful situations. This can be positive stress, such as running a marathon or interviewing for a job. It can also be negative stress, such as being stuck in traffic on the way to the job interview.

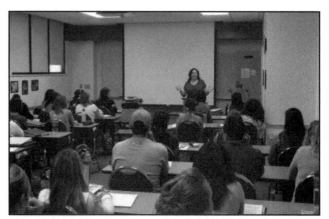

Figure 5-30. Giving a speech may challenge heart rate and blood pressure.

Heart Rate

The function of the heart is to deliver blood to all areas of the body. The rate at which this occurs (how often the heart contracts) is based on the need for blood and oxygen to areas of the body. Thus, the heart will need to pump faster when there is a higher demand, such as when extremities are moving and require blood and oxygen to function. There are many factors that can contribute to a change in heart rate, including the autonomic nervous system and adrenaline. Typically, during activity the heart rate should not exceed 20 beats per minute above the resting heart rate. Maintaining the heart rate needed to deliver the appropriate amount of blood and oxygen to the body is a function that is often challenged during activities that require a great amount of movement or varied amounts of movement where the heart rate may need to fluctuate between high and low. Activities that challenge heart rate may also be those that stimulate the sympathetic nervous system through stressful situations. For example, when taking an exam or meeting someone you are attracted to, your heart rate may increase.

Having a heart that beats on a consistent basis is a necessity of living; however, the extent to which maintenance or obtaining a specific heart rate is required of an activity relies upon the context in which the activity occurs. The amount of physical challenge to the body will determine the amount by which the heart rate will need to increase to meet the circulatory demands of the body. Does the activity require the starting and stopping of movement and thus the heart needing to regulate the rate in which it is pumping from slow to fast and then return to a resting heart rate? Is there a psychological stressor involved in the activity that may challenge the heart to increase the rate at which it is beating?

Hematological and Immunological Systems Functions

Hematological System

The hematological system relates to the blood and the blood-forming tissues of the body which include the bone marrow and spleen (*Mosby's Dictionary*, 2006). The primary function of blood is to carry oxygen and nutrients to cells within the body. Blood also carries away carbon dioxide and other wastes to be removed from the body. It is our blood that transports hormones that signal other areas of the body into action. Blood also allows wounds to stop bleeding and send an immunological defense to fight infections. The hematological system is essential for survival and is challenged during activities that require efficient delivery of certain elements to parts of the body. An example of this would be delivery of electrolytes to muscles used during a physically strenuous activity. It is also required if there is risk of bruising or injury. If contact with objects occurs, the clotting functions of the blood allow physical contact with objects or other people that may cause bruising or abrasions without continuous bleeding.

Immunological System

The immune system works to protect the body against infection and other pathological organisms and actions. The immune system is composed of the bone marrow, thymus, spleen, and lymph tissues (*Mosby's Dictionary*, 2006). Immunology, the study of body's response to threats, is a complex and expansive area of human science. For the sake of activity analysis, the OT practitioner needs to have a basic understanding of how the immune system plays a role in the engagement in activities. There are practitioners who specialize in this area and develop a deeper understanding of how the function or dysfunction of the immune system can influence participation in occupations. An example of this is a practitioner who specializes in lymphedema management. In this area of practice, the clinician works with clients who are limited by an excessive accumulation of lymph fluid in a limb.

The immunological system is utilized in everyday activities, to a greater extent when confronted with environments that present hazards. For example, if sitting inside our own home reading a book, our immune systems are not challenged. However, if playing on the playground with other children, our immune systems must go to work to fight off the multiple viruses and bacteria we may be exposed to. When analyzing an activity and determining if the immune system is challenged, think about the environment in which the activity commonly occurs. Does the activity occur outside of the person's home? Is there interaction with others? Does the person need to touch objects that have been touched by others or have been outdoors? How clean is the typical environment?

Additional Functions and Sensations of the Cardiovascular and Respiratory Systems

Rate of Respiration

Respiration is the process of moving air in and out of the lungs. The rate in which this occurs typically ranges from 12 to 20 breaths per minute in adults (*Mosby's Dictionary*, 2006). The rate in which air is brought into the lungs is dependent upon the body's need for oxygen. Because oxygen is required for movement of the body, with increased movement there is an increased demand for oxygen. Thus, for activities that require great amounts of movement, the respiration rate increases to meet the demands. Slower rates of respiration may be required for activities focused on relaxation or sleep. The amount of oxygen available in the air may influence the rate of respiration as experienced in higher elevations. When the air in the environment contains a lower concentration of oxygen, the lungs must work harder to supply a sufficient amount of oxygen to the body. Thus, activities conducted at higher elevations will require a greater challenge to respiratory rate.

Rhythm of Respiration

Respiratory rhythm is the cycle of inspiration and expiration of air from the lungs (*Mosby's Dictionary*, 2006). A normal breathing pattern will match the demands for oxygen in the body. Abnormal rhythms are seen when there is a brief cessation of breathing when there is a need for oxygen in the body, rapid cycles when at rest, or ataxic breathing where there are quick breaths alternating with slow ones. The demand for a specific rhythm of respiration increases as the demands for oxygen change. As a person starts to move or stops moving, the rhythm in which he or she is breathing should change accordingly. In activities where there is continuous movement, a respiratory rate that will allow the body to continue moving efficiently must be established. An example of this is with long-distance running. Experienced runners learn to pattern their respirations so that they

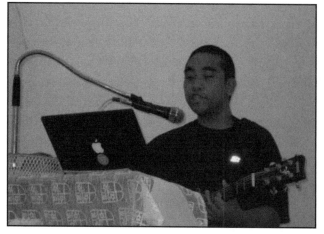

Figure 5-31. The rhythm of respiration is challenged while singing.

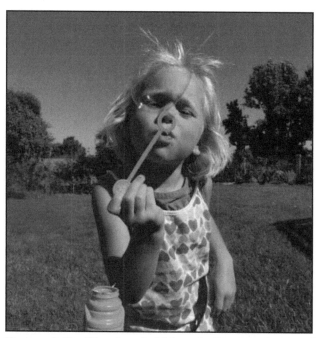

Figure 5-32. Blowing bubbles challenges depth of respiration.

are breathing efficiently. The rhythm of respiration is challenged in other activities such as swimming, where there is a cessation of breathing for periods of time, followed by a large inhale. Rhythm of respiration is also challenged during singing (Figure 5-31) or delivering a speech. Activities that involve production of speech or sounds via the mouth will include controlling respiratory rhythm. Eating also requires regulating the rhythm of respiration around swallowing of foods and liquids.

Depth of Respiration

Depth of respiration refers to the volume of air inhaled and exhaled (WHO, 2001). Shallow breathing occurs when small amounts of air are inhaled. Smaller amounts produce smaller amounts of oxygen distributed to the body. The depth of respiration is linked to the need for oxygen in other areas of the body. With greater demands for oxygen, respiration depth is greater. For example, if climbing a tree, our lungs will expand and inhale deeper than when we are sitting and reading a book. The depth of inspiration can also be influenced by what we will be doing with the exhalation. Singing or playing a musical instrument such as a flute will require a deep inspiration, as the long and sustained exhalation will be utilized to create music.

To determine the extent to which this function is utilized, think about how much the body is moving. Does the body move over a period of time in which blood will need to deliver adequate oxygen? This means that a simple short movement such as reaching for a book may not require deep respirations, but repeating this motion repeatedly would. Does the activity require use of air coming out of the body,

such as blowing up a balloon, blowing bubbles (Figure 5-32), whistling, singing, or playing a wind instrument?

Physical Endurance, Stamina, Aerobic Capacity

Endurance as it relates to the cardiovascular and respiratory systems involves continuous efficient action of the heart and lungs to provide oxygen to the body. Cardiac endurance requires that the heart maintain a rate and rhythm over time as the body moves throughout the activity. This is essential for activities that occur over a longer period of time with few breaks. This means that the heart and lungs must endure a certain pace and provide the necessary oxygen to the rest of the body as needed. It is this cardiac and respiratory endurance that often challenges many people during aerobic exercise. Not only is muscle endurance required but also the endurance of the heart and lungs to provide oxygen to those muscles.

Activities that utilize physical endurance and stamina require prolonged movement and increased respiratory and heart rates. Activities that require continuous movement with little to no rest breaks will challenge this factor. When analyzing an activity to determine if physical endurance is utilized, think about how much the person must stand or move. Are there any opportunities for break, when the heart

Activity 5-9

REVIEW OF CARDIOVASCULAR, HEMATOLOGICAL, IMMUNOLOGICAL, AND RESPIRATORY FUNCTIONS

Identify how each of the following functions is utilized while buying a snack out of a vending machine. Assume that you are already standing in front of the machine with change in your pants pocket. Leave a row blank if a factor is not used. In the final columns, indicate the extent to which each body function is challenged during this activity.

Function	How It Is Used	None	Minimally Challenged	Greatly Challenged
Blood pressure				
Heart rate				
Respiratory rate				
Respiratory rhythm				
Respiratory depth				
Physical endurance, aerobic capacity				

rate and respiratory rate will have a chance to lower to close to a resting rate? Are the heart and lungs required to maintain a particular rate for a prolonged period of time, such as in singing or swimming?

The ICF defines aerobic capacity as "the extent to which a person can exercise without getting out of breath" (WHO, 2001, p. 80). Reaching the point of being out of breath is determined by the efficiency in which the body is utilizing oxygen. When the body is not able to absorb and utilize the appropriate amount of oxygen needed, the body's natural reaction is to increase the respiration rate to increase the amount of oxygen the lungs are bringing into the body. Thus, aerobic capacity is about the amount of physiologic work the body must do in order to absorb oxygen. An activity that requires a high level of aerobic capacity is one that requires the body to efficiently absorb oxygen while moving for long periods of time. Aerobic capacity is required of all activities that require long periods of movement and require sufficient delivery of oxygen to the limbs or muscles used. Hiking and long-distance bicycling are examples of when aerobic capacity is challenged.

Use Activity 5-9 as a review for this section.

SECTION 5: VOICE AND SPEECH, DIGESTIVE, METABOLIC, ENDOCRINE, GENITOURINARY, REPRODUCTIVE, SKIN, AND RELATED STRUCTURE FUNCTIONS

Voice and Speech Functions

Voice Functions

Voice functions are those that produce noise by sending air through the larynx (WHO, 2001). Humans use this noise that is produced as a primary mode of communication—speech. Without voice, our mouths would move but nothing would be heard. Producing a voice requires a coordination of the respiratory system and the larynx and surrounding muscles. This coordination is what allows for volume, pitch, and resonance of a voice (WHO, 2001). Identifying the need for this function in activity is fairly easy, in that if any talking is involved, then it is needed. The extent to which this factor is challenged depends on the extent to which the voice is utilized—at what volume, at various pitches, and with what quality. Delivering a speech is an activity that requires a high level of voice functions, whereas an activity that requires a low level would be talking face to face with a friend or whispering to the person next to you in class.

Rhythm and Fluency

In order to be understood by others when we speak, a certain flow and tempo is used to express the beginning and ending of statements, emotion, and emphasis on specific words. For example, when telling a joke, the punch line is usually told with a certain intonation that indicates to the listener that those last few words are the highlight of the joke. The rhythm of our speech patterns also communicates to the listener the emotion behind what is being said. Rapid speech sends a message of urgency, while slow, deliberate speech communicates a more relaxed feeling (Figure 5-33).

Fluency is what allows us to smoothly speak one word after another fluidly and smoothly. Without this, we would stumble over words or repeat parts of words, as is seen in stuttering. Being able to smoothly transition from one word to another is what allows us to communicate efficiently and effectively. This is especially important when trying to portray an urgent message or communicating to those we do not know. For example, if calling a 911 operator, it is imperative that we be able to fluently and smoothly string together the words needed to communicate what emergency is occurring. Rhythm and fluency are utilized when producing speech but challenged when confronted with activities with higher social demands. When the expectations or needs of the listener are higher, the demand for rhythm and fluency increases.

Alternative Vocalization Functions

There are times in which vocalizations are produced for activities outside of those involving speaking. Alternative vocalizations are those needed for yelling, singing, humming, chanting, or crying. Before we gain the ability to speak, crying is the human's way of communicating. Even after learning how to speak, we continue to use alternative vocalizations for calling attention to others—by yelling. Singing, humming, and chanting are sustained vocalizations that produce noise but do not necessarily entail the use of words.

Activities that require alternative vocalizations are those in which typical speech is not utilized but the vocal cords are still used. Children and infants

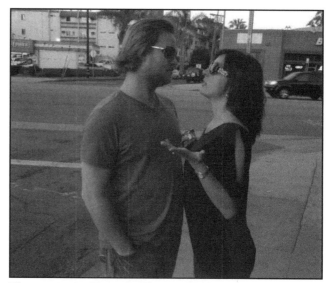

Figure 5-33. Voice and speech functions are challenged in communicating to others.

utilize this function in much of what they do during waking hours. Adults may communicate with infants in similar ways with coos and babbles. Laughter is considered an alternative vocalization that is utilized in many activities throughout the lifespan. These alternative vocalizations are still a means by which to communicate; it is simply doing so without the use of forming words. Activities that utilize this function are those that demand or produce some use of the voice during the course of the activity. Children and infants will require this function as a way to communicate needs; when they are hungry or have a dirty diaper, they will produce a cry. Communicating to others a sense of joy or happiness during an activity will require this function to produce a laugh or giggle. In situations where the attention of another or perhaps an animal is required, a loud noise or yell will be needed.

Digestive, Metabolic, and Endocrine Systems Functions

Digestive System Function

The digestive system is what allows for transportation of food or liquids through the body to be absorbed and broken down (WHO, 2001). When food is swallowed, it moves through the gastrointestinal system by movements called *peristalsis*. Peristalsis moves the food from the stomach and into the intestines. While it is in each area of the gastrointestinal system, nutrients are absorbed from the food into the body. Activities that include eating or drinking will require the digestive system. Greater challenges to the system will be meals of greater size and complexity. For example, food items that are more difficult to digest (i.e., are denser in consistency) will be a greater challenge to the digestive system.

Metabolic System

The metabolic system is what allows our bodies to utilize food and convert it to energy. This includes the breakdown and utilization of carbohydrates, proteins, and fats (WHO, 2001). This broad and basic definition does not fairly reveal the complexity of this system. However, the *Framework* states that as OT practitioners, we are to have a broad understanding of how this function influences engagement in occupation. As mentioned earlier, there are clinicians that may choose to specialize in some of these functions, necessitating extra training and education. On a basic level, the metabolic system is utilized when the body needs to utilize food as energy. The greater amount of energy needed, the greater demand on the metabolic system to perform. For example, swimming requires energy supplied to the arms and legs in order to allow the muscles to contract. Without a source of energy, the muscles would be unable to move the limbs.

Endocrine System

Much like the metabolic system, the endocrine system is complex and will get little time in the spotlight here, and will require further inquiry for those involved in this specialty area. The endocrine system regulates hormone levels within the body, including growth and metabolic hormones (*Mosby's Dictionary*, 2006; WHO, 2001). The glands and other structures that secrete hormones help regulate daily, monthly, and annual rhythms. These hormones are often what drive us toward certain actions and allow us to function day to day. It is what gives us drive toward reproduction, controls appetite, and allows mothers to produce milk while nursing their babies. Some hormones regulate the salt and water balance in the body when engaging in strenuous activity. These are just a few of the ways the endocrine system is utilized in activities beyond keeping the human body alive and healthy. Refer to endocrinology literature for a greater understanding of the scope of this system.

Genitourinary and Reproductive Functions

Urinary Functions

Urinary functions are utilized for one purpose only—to release urine from the body (WHO, 2001).

This includes controlling the release of the urine, which is called *continence*. The ability to refrain from releasing urine at inappropriate times is required for most activities, especially those around other people. This function is especially challenged when the person is required to go long periods of time before being able to urinate. An example of this might be if riding in a bicycle race. There would be minimal opportunity to relieve the bladder along the long trail. Urinary functions are especially in demand when urination is part of the activity, such as when using the bathroom or if giving a urine sample while visiting the doctor. To determine the extent to which urinary functions are required of an activity, think about the context(s) in which the activity occurs and if there is opportunity to empty the bladder. How much time passes between the opportunities for this? Is the person required to hold his or her urine for long periods of time? Is urination part of the activity? Are there social demands of the activity that require the person be continent? Certainly a person in front of an audience must not relieve him- or herself while giving a speech.

Genital and Reproductive Functions

According to the ICF, the genital and reproductive functions include sexual functions, menstruation, procreation, and sensations associated with genital and reproductive functions (WHO, 2001). Sexual functions are related to the mental and physical aspects of performing sexual acts (WHO, 2001). These acts do not necessarily require the involvement of another person. The menstrual cycle is also controlled by the reproductive system and regulates the regularity and extent of menstrual bleeding. Of course, this occurrence is only experienced by women. The ability to procreate or create and give birth to a child is also part of the genital and reproductive functions. Male and female fertility is required in order to create a fetus, followed by the woman's ability to carry the child in her uterus until birth. It is the genital and reproductive functions that give women the ability to produce milk for the child once born.

Activities that require genital and reproductive functions will be those that involve sexual activity that incorporates the genitals. The genitals can be used for creating a child or for enjoyment only. If the purpose of sexual activity is to procreate, the demands on this function are greater, as fertility functions will be required. Any activity surrounding the menstrual cycle will also require this function, as with some self-care activities.

Skin and Related Structure Functions

Protective Functions of the Skin

The skin is designed to protect us from physical, chemical, and biological elements that might cause harm to our bodies (WHO, 2001). This is especially important when surrounded by or coming in contact with elements that, if they gain access to our blood stream, would cause us harm. Our hands come in contact with bacteria and germs on a continuous basis, but the skin surrounding our fingers prevents these from entering our bodies. Protection fails when these elements are introduced to our mouths, nose, or cuts in the skin. The elements of the environment such as wind, heat, cold, and sun are also shielded by our skin. Environments that experience extreme temperatures or climates challenge the protective functions of the skin to work hard.

Any time we come in contact with an object or other person, the protective functions of our skin are utilized to protect us. The greater the amount of pressure or shearing forces, the greater the challenge is to this function. For example, if shoveling dirt in a garden, the skin on the hands is challenged to endure the shearing forces of the shovel handle against the skin. The environment is also a consideration in analyzing the extent to which this function is utilized. Is there extreme heat where the skin is required to sweat? Is the skin exposed to sun or wind? Extreme conditions will challenge the skin to protect the inner temperature of the body.

Repair Function of the Skin–Wound Healing

Skin has the amazing capacity to heal itself. When damage occurs through tearing, ripping, cutting, or burning, the skin begins a process of repairing the wound. This process is required of activities in which maintaining skin integrity is important. As mentioned in the previous section, the skin serves to protect the human body; without such it is at risk for exposure to harmful elements. If an activity involves the chance of injury to the skin, the repair functions of the skin will be necessary. Activities that require a person to regain skin integrity in order to continue on with an

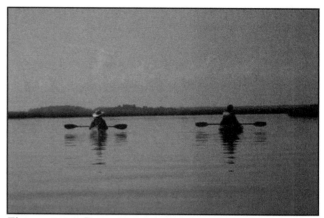

Figure 5-34. Repetitive motions such as rowing challenge the skin functions of the hands.

activity will also utilize this function. An example of this would be the activity of participating on a rowing team. If a blister develops on the rower's hand, his or her wound-healing functions must quickly go to work to allow the person to get back to rowing on the team (Figure 5-34).

Use Activity 5-10 as a review for this section.

CONCLUSION

The *Framework* delineates that part of determining the demands of an activity include examining the body functions required. Body functions are the physiological aspects of the human body such as sensory, mental, neuromuscular, skeletal, and cardiovascular functions. Body functions are the features that reside within the client that influence skill level but do not assure a certain skill level. Skill level is influenced by many factors such as the environment and the challenges of the activity. Engagement in an activity requires a complex interaction of many body functions. Activity analysis includes understanding the role of each of the body functions and the extent to which each is challenged during an activity. With this knowledge, the clinician can better understand what contributes or limits participation in occupations and can be used to develop strategies for intervention (Activity 5-11).

Activity 5-10

REVIEW OF VOICE AND SPEECH, DIGESTIVE, METABOLIC, ENDOCRINE, GENITOURINARY, REPRODUCTIVE, SKIN, AND RELATED STRUCTURE FUNCTIONS

Identify how each of the following functions is utilized while buying a snack out of a vending machine. Assume that you are already standing in front of the machine with change in your pants pocket. Leave a row blank if a factor is not used. In the final columns, indicate the extent to which each body function is challenged during this activity.

Function	How It Is Used	None	Minimally Challenged	Greatly Challenged
Voice functions				
Voice rhythm and fluency				
Alternative vocalization				
Digestive system				
Metabolic system				
Endocrine system				
Urinary functions				
Genital and reproductive function				
Protective functions of the skin				
Repair functions of the skin				

QUESTIONS

1. What is the difference between judgment and cognitive flexibility?

2. In what activities is insight an important body function?

3. What is multisensory processing and why is it important?

4. Of the perceptual functions, which do you utilize the most when driving? When studying? When grocery shopping?

5. Which of the thought functions do you utilize the most when driving, studying, or grocery shopping?

6. What is the difference between emotional stability and coping?

7. Why would tolerance of ambient sounds be needed during activities?

8. Describe the function of awareness of body and space and how it is utilized. How is it different from moving securely against gravity?

9. What is muscle tone?

10. In what populations would you see ATNR and STNR?

11. Name five activities that require bilateral integration.

12. In what types of activities would alternative vocalization functions be utilized?

Activity 5-11

Determine the body functions required of washing hair in the shower as it typically is done. Describe briefly how each of the body functions is used and then indicate the extent to which each body function is challenged. If a body function is not used at all during the activity, check off "none" and leave that row blank.

Function	How It Is Used	None	Minimally Challenged	Greatly Challenged
Judgment				
Concept formation				
Metacognition				
Cognitive flexibility				
Insight/awareness				
Sustained attention				
Selective attention				
Divided attention				
Short-term memory				
Working memory				
Long-term memory				
Discrimination of senses: Auditory				
Discrimination of senses: Tactile				
Discrimination of senses: Visual				
Discrimination of senses: Olfactory				
Discrimination of senses: Vestibular-proprioception				
Multisensory processing				
Sensory memory				
Spatial relationships				
Temporal relationships				
Recognition				
Categorization				
Generalization				
Awareness of reality				
Logical/coherent thought				
Appropriate thought content				
Execution of learned movements				
Coping				
Behavioral regulation				
Body image				
Self-concept				
Self-esteem				
Arousal				
Consciousness				
Orientation to self				

(continued)

Activity 5-11 (continued)

Function	How It Is Used	None	Minimally Challenged	Greatly Challenged
Orientation to place				
Orientation to time				
Orientation to others				
Emotional stability				
Motivation				
Impulse control				
Appetite				
Sleep				
Detection/registration				
Visual modulation				
Integration of senses				
Awareness at distances				
Tolerance of ambient sounds				
Location and distance of sounds				
Moving against gravity				
Taste				
Smell				
Body and space				
Comfort with touch				
Localizing pain				
Thermal awareness				
Joint range of motion				
Joint stability/alignment				
Strength				
Muscle tone				
Muscle endurance				
Stretch reflex				
ATNR				
STNR				
Righting and supporting reflex				
Eye–hand coordination				
Eye–foot coordination				
Bilateral coordination				
Crossing midline				
Fine motor control				
Gross motor control				
Oculomotor control				
Gait patterns				
Blood pressure				
Heart rate				
Respiratory rate				
Respiratory rhythm				

(continued)

Function	How It Is Used	None	Minimally Challenged	Greatly Challenged
Respiratory depth				
Physical endurance, aerobic capacity				
Voice functions				
Voice fluency and rhythm				
Alternative vocalization				
Digestive system				
Metabolic system				
Endocrine system				
Urinary functions				
Genital and reproductive function				
Protective functions of the skin				
Repair functions of the skin				

REFERENCES

Al-Hilawani, Y. (2003). Measuring students' metacognition in real life situations. *American Annals of the Deaf, 148*(3), 233–242.

Al-Hilawani, Y., Easterbrooks, S., & Marchant, G. (2002). Metacognitive ability from a theory of mind perspective: A cross-cultural study of students with and without hearing loss. *American Annals of the Deaf, 147,* 38–47.

American Occupational Therapy Association. (2008). Occupational therapy practice framework: Domain and process (2nd ed.). *American Journal of Occupational Therapy, 62,* 625–683.

Barco, P., Grosson, B., Bolesta, M., Werts, D., & Stout, R. (1991). *Cognitive rehabilitation for persons with traumatic brain injury.* Baltimore, MD: Paul H. Brooks Publishing.

Barnard, C. (1995). Mind in everyday affairs: An examination into logical and non-logical thought processes. *Journal of Management History, 1,* 7–28.

Bolding, D., Adler, C., Tipton-Burton, M. & Lillie, S. (2009). Mobility. In E. Crepeau, E. Cohn, & B. Boyt Schell (Eds.), *Willard and Spackman's occupational therapy* (11th ed., pp. 195–247). Philadelphia, PA: Lippincott Williams & Wilkins.

Breines, E. (2009). Therapeutic occupations and modalities. In H. Pendleton & W. Schultz-Krohn (Eds.), *Pedretti's occupational therapy. Practice skills for physical dysfunction* (pp. 658–679). St. Louis, MO: Mosby Elsevier.

Brown, A. (1978). Knowing when, where, and how to remember: A problem of metacognition. In R. Glaser (Ed.), *Advances in instructional psychology* (pp. 55–113). Hillsdale, NJ: Erlbaum.

Buckley, K., & Poole, S. (2004). Activity analysis. In H. Hinojosa & M. Blount (Eds.), *The texture of life* (pp. 69–114). Bethesda, MD: AOTA Press.

Bukowski, E. (2000). *Muscular analysis of everyday activities.* Thorofare, NJ: SLACK Incorporated.

Cooper, C., & Abrams, M. (2006). Evaluation of sensation and intervention for sensory dysfunction. In H. Pendleton & W. Schultz-Krohn (Eds.), *Pedretti's occupational therapy. Practice skills for physical dysfunction* (pp. 513–531). St. Louis, MO: Mosby Elsevier.

Crosson, C., Barco, P., Velozo, C., Bolesta, M., Cooper, P., & Werts, D. (1989). Awareness and compensation in post-acute head injury rehabilitation. *Journal of Clinical and Experimental Neuropsychology, 2,* 355–363.

de Bruin, A. (2008). Evaluation of vestibular proprioceptive (VPP) functioning in children: Identification of relevant test items. *South African Journal of Occupational Therapy, 38*(3), 14–17.

Dunn, W. (2009). Sensation and sensory processing. In E. Crepeau, E. Cohn, & B. Boyt Schell (Eds.), *Willard and Spackman's occupational therapy,* (11th ed., pp. 777–791). Philadelphia, PA: Lippincott Williams & Wilkins.

Flavell, J. (1979). Metacognition and cognitive monitoring: A new era in psychological inquiry. *American Psychologist, 34,* 906–911.

Levy, B., & Dreier, T. (1997). Preservation of temporal skills in Alzheimer's disease, *Perception and Motor Skills, 85,* 83–96.

Levy, L. (2005). Cognitive aging in perspective: Information processing, cognition and memory. In N. Katz (Ed.), *Cognition and occupation across the life span* (2nd ed., pp. 305–325). Bethesda, MD: American Occupational Therapy Association.

Mosby's dictionary of medicine, nursing & health professions. (2006). St. Louis, MO: Mosby Elsevier.

Munguba, M., Valdes, M., & Da Silva, C. (2008). The application of an occupational therapy nutrition education programme for children who are obese. *Occupational Therapy International, 15*(1), 56–70.

Parente, R., & Anderson, J. (1991). *Retraining memory: Techniques and applications.* Houston, TX: CSY Publishing.

Parker, R. (1990). *Traumatic brain injury and neuropsychological impairment.* New York, NY: Springer-Verlag.

Preston, L. (2009). Evaluation of motor control. In H. Pendleton & W. Schultz-Krohn (Eds.), *Pedretti's occupational therapy. Practice skills for physical dysfunction* (pp. 403–428). St. Louis, MO: Mosby Elsevier.

Pizur-Barnekow, K., Kraemer, G., & Winters, J. (2008). Pilot study investigating infant vagal reactivity and visual behavior during object perception. *American Journal of Occupational Therapy, 62*(2), 198–205.

Rahman, R., & Sommer, W. (2008). Seeing what we know and understand: How knowledge shapes perception. *Psychonomic Bulliten and Review, 15*(6), 1055–1064.

Roley, S., & Jacobs, S. E. (2009). Sensory integration. In E. Crepeau, E. Cohn, & B. Boyt Schell (Eds.), *Willard and Spackman's occupational therapy* (11th ed., pp. 792–817). Philadelphia, PA: Lippincott Williams & Wilkins.

Shams, L., Kamitani, Y., & Shimojo, S. (2004). Modulations of visual perception by sound. In G. Calvert, C. Spence, & B.E. Stein (Eds.), *The handbook of multisensory processes* (pp. 27–34). Cambridge, MA: MIT Press.

Warren, M. (2009). Evaluation and treatment of visual deficits following brain injury. In E. Crepeau, E. Cohn, & B. Boyt Schell (Eds.), *Willard and Spackman's occupational therapy* (11th ed., pp. 532–572). Philadelphia, PA: Lippincott Williams & Wilkins.

White, B. (2009). Psychobiological factors. In E. Crepeau, E. Cohn, & B. Boyt Schell (Eds.), *Willard and Spackman's occupational therapy* (11th ed., pp. 716–738). Philadelphia, PA: Lippincott Williams & Wilkins.

World Health Organization. (2001). *International classification of functioning, disability, and health.* Geneva, Switzerland: Author.

Zemke, R. (1994). Task skills, problem solving, and social interaction. In C. B. Royeen (Ed.), *AOTA self study series: Cognitive rehabilitation.* Bethesda, MD: American Occupational Therapy Association

Zoltan, B. (2007). *Vision, perception, and cognition* (4th ed.). Thorofare, NJ: SLACK Incorporated.

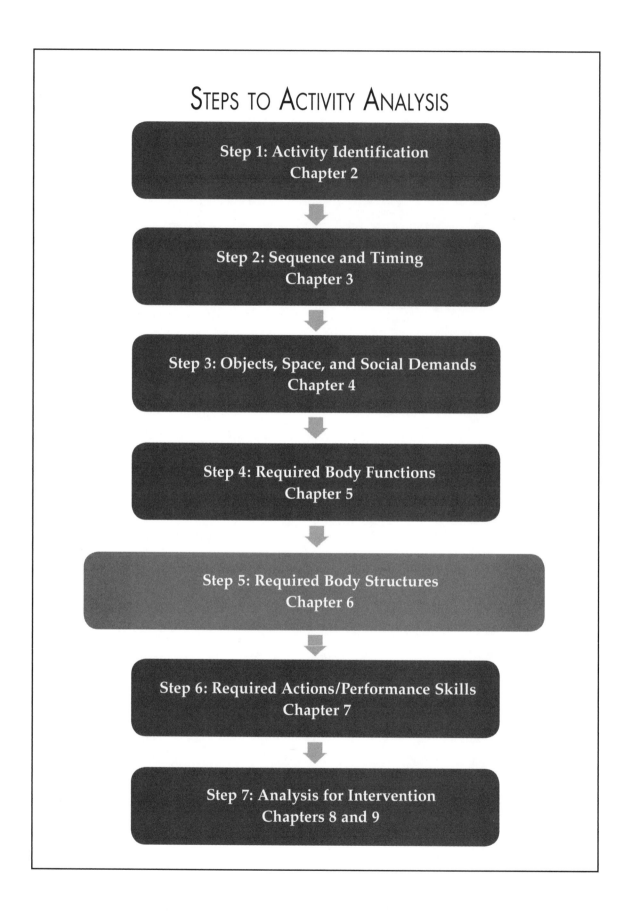

6

REQUIRED BODY STRUCTURES

OBJECTIVES

1. Define what body structures are according to the *Occupational Therapy Practice Framework, 2nd Edition (Framework)*.

2. Identify the steps to determining the body structures required of an activity.

3. Understand why occupational therapy (OT) practitioners need to have a basic understanding of how body structures influence performance in activities.

4. Define the body structures included in the nervous, eyes, ears, voice and speech, cardiovascular, immune, respiratory, digestive, metabolic, endocrine, genitourinary, and reproductive systems as well as movement and skin-related structures.

5. Identify the body functions influenced by each specific body structure.

6. Understand how body systems work collaboratively to meet the demands of activities.

Body structures are those anatomical parts that support body functions (American Occupational Therapy Association [AOTA], 2008). This includes the limbs, organs, and structures of each organ. For example, to allow a person to use his or her respiratory functions to breathe at the needed rate, the structure of the lungs and circulatory system must work efficiently and be intact in order to support respiratory functions. Each of the body functions listed in the *Framework* is supported by one or more

body structure systems. The *Framework* utilizes the classification of body systems which is used by the World Health Organization (WHO) in the *International Classification of Functioning, Disability, and Health* (ICF). There are eight broad categories, some of which have several systems categorized together.

Instead of defining each of the body structures, the *Framework* refers the reader to the ICF classifications and states:

> *Occupational therapy practitioners have knowledge of body structures and understand broadly the interaction that occurs between these structures to support health and participation in life through engagement in occupation. Some therapists may specialize in evaluating and intervening with a specific structure as it is related to supporting performance and engagement in occupations and activities targeted for intervention.* (AOTA, 2008, p. 637).

It is assumed that through entry-level OT education, the clinician gains a basic understanding of the different body systems and how they contribute to engaging in daily activities. The structure of body systems influences body functions and is thus part of the demands of engagement in activity. Part of analyzing an activity is understanding how the body systems are required of the activity being analyzed. Identifying the extent to which each body *function* is utilized, which you learned how to do in the last chapter, will help in determining which body structures are required of an activity. Body structures support body functions and thus, by identifying the functions, you will be able to identify the structures

Thomas, H. *Occupation-Based Activity Analysis* (pp. 107-123).
© 2012 SLACK Incorporated

needed. For example, by looking at the list of body functions required of washing hair in the shower, we will see that the sensation of touch is used to feel the soap suds and where the hair is as it is being washed. The touch receptors that are in the tips of the fingers receive information from what is being touched and send an electrical signal along nerves that run up the arm to the spinal cord, and then from the spinal cord to the brain. In the brain, the signal is interpreted. All of these anatomical structures are required in order to sense what is being touched. The lack of or damage to a part of the structure can cause deficiencies in functioning. As we examine the different body structure systems, the body functions that rely on that structure system will be identified and the connection between the two will become more evident.

While identifying the body functions required is a good way to begin distinguishing which body structures are needed, some are required of an activity even though they do not support a body function. This is true when a particular part of the body interacts with elements of the environment or actions that occur or is used in conjunction with objects used in the activity. An example of this is with the cranial bones, which are part of the structures related to movement. These are the bones that enclose the brain, making up the skull. These hard bones serve to protect the brain from impact from external forces. These bones will be very necessary when engaging in occupations in which the head comes in contact with objects, such as a soccer ball when playing soccer. Another example is when eyelids and eyebrows are used when communicating (i.e., winking or raising the eyebrows in expression of emotion). So, when analyzing an activity for the needed body structures, think about what body parts are used during the activity, as well as the body functions that need support from body structures.

Steps to identifying required body structures:

+ Match the body functions that are needed with the supporting body structures.

+ Identify which body parts are used during the activity.

+ Determine which parts of the body come in contact with external forces.

The following sections give a brief description of each of the body structure systems that the *Framework* has identified, along with the ICF definition of what structures make up that system. Each structure that is listed has corresponding body functions that it supports. While this presents an introduction to each of the systems as it relates to engagement in occupations, further reading is recommended for a more in-depth understanding of particular body systems.

STRUCTURES OF THE NERVOUS SYSTEM

The brain is the central structure of the nervous system, processing both sensory information and sending motor responses. It is the brain and the corresponding structure that control all thought processes and thinking skills. The function of the nervous system and each of the structures is complex, to which volumes of texts and courses are dedicated. The following is a brief introduction to the basic functions of each of the structures.

The structures of the brain include the lobes of the brain, midbrain, cerebellum, brainstem, and cranial nerves. There are four lobes of the brain: occipital, temporal, frontal, and parietal. The primary function of the occipital lobe is to process visual information. The temporal lobe controls learning, memory, language, and auditory information. The frontal lobe is involved in movement, judgment, emotional behavior, problem solving, and language expression. The parietal lobe controls the processing of visuospatial and somatosensory (sensations from the body) information, as well as interpreting language (Loma Linda University, 2004). The midbrain, or the mesencephalon, is a relay center for visual and auditory information, and controls eye and bodily movements (*Mosby's Dictionary*, 2006). The diencephalon, which is composed of the thalamus, hypothalamus, subthalamus, and epithalamus, is a small but essential hub for many functions of the brain. The diencephalon has a role in sleep, sensation, movement, cognition, emotion, and arousal. It also serves as a sensory relay station for information sent to the brain regarding information received from the sensory systems. The hypothalamus, which is part of the diencephalon, controls autonomic, endocrine, and emotional functions (Filley, 2002). The basal ganglia controls the subconscious modulation of movements, especially organizing movements as to prevent tremors (Crosson, Maron, Moore, & Grande, 2002). When this area of the brain is impaired, as occurs in Parkinson's disease, muscular tremors are uncontrollable. The cerebellum is primarily responsible for coordination, postural control, equilibrium, and muscle tone (Molinari, 2002).

The brainstem controls many essential functions of the body. This includes sleep/wake cycles, consciousness, pupil size, voluntary and involuntary movement of the eyes, body movement, posture, touch, temperature, pain, hearing, moving against gravity, taste, salivating, chewing and swallowing, gastrointestinal functions, urination, breathing, blood flow/pressure, and cardiac functions (Blessing, 2002). There are 12 cranial nerves that provide sensory and motor neural transmission for the head and neck.

Structurally, they are connected to the brain and are thus considered structures of the brain. Each of the cranial nerves sends and receives messages for specific functions including smell, vision, eye movement, sensations of the head and face, chewing, hearing, balance, movement of the tongue, taste, and swallow functions (Butler, 2002). Table 6-1 describes which body functions are reliant on each of the different structures of the brain.

The structures of the spinal cord also serve a purpose in the nervous system, as a relay for sensory and motor signals. The spinal cord contains nerves that travel from the base of the brain through the spinal column (which is protected by bony vertebrae) and down to the bottom of the spinal column. The cord works as a conduit for messages being sent to and from the body. Structures within the spinal cord also control reflexive actions as well, bypassing the brain. From the spinal cord branch 31 pairs of spinal nerves which extend out to all areas of the body, each pair emerging from one of the 31 vertebrae (Walker & Parker, 2009). The spinal nerves that emerge at each level of vertebrae control and send neural impulses from a different area of the body. Each set of spinal nerves is named according to the level of the vertebral column from which they emerge. Thus, there are eight cervical, 12 thoracic, five lumbar, five sacral, and one coccygeal pairs. In each pair, there are posterior roots that are primarily sensory neurons and ventral (anterior) roots that contain motor neurons (*Mosby's Dictionary*, 2006). It is through these spinal nerves that sensation and motor movement is controlled.

The meninges are the three membranes that encompass and protect the spinal cord and brain. The sympathetic nervous system automatically prepares the body for emergency or stressful situations, while the parasympathetic nervous systems works to restore the body to a more relaxed state. In the face of danger or stress, the sympathetic nervous system causes the pupils to dilate, the bronchial tubes to open, the heart rate to increase, and stomach digestive functions to slow. As the danger or stressor is removed, the parasympathetic nervous system constricts the pupils and bronchial tubes, decreases the heart rate, and restores digestion (Walker & Parker, 2009) (See Table 6-1).

EYES, EARS, AND RELATED STRUCTURES

The structures of the eye are those that allow visual data to be sent to the brain for interpretation of information. Without intact structures within and around the eye, images may be distorted or unable to be interpreted. This includes the structures that make up the eyeball itself, as well as the structures that surround it and contribute to sight. The same is true of the ear and the structures that allow for hearing. There are external, middle, and inner ear structures that work in conjunction with each other to allow for reception of sounds, as well as position in space (See Table 6-2).

STRUCTURES INVOLVED IN VOICE AND SPEECH

There are several parts of the body that control the ability to speak. Typically, the larynx is thought of as the primary structure involved in speech, but in order to form words and project the sounds, the structures of the nose, mouth, and pharynx are also required. The body functions reliant on these structures are only the voice and speech functions (See Table 6-3).

STRUCTURES OF THE CARDIOVASCULAR, IMMUNOLOGICAL, AND RESPIRATORY SYSTEMS

The ICF and *Framework* lump these three major body systems together. While each of them serves a very specific function, all of them are essential to maintaining human life. The next set of body structures and related body function tables divide each of the systems separately so that it is evident what each of these provides (See Tables 6-4 to 6-7). Each of these systems is reliant upon each other and contributes to the existence and survival of other systems. For example, without adequate circulation, the neurological systems would be ineffective. It is with this assumption that the circulatory, respiratory, and immunological systems are not listed as required of all of the body functions, as it is assumed they are required for human life. When analyzing an activity for the body system requirements in this area, think about what body functions are challenged, which in turn challenge the corresponding body structures.

Cardiovascular System

The heart's atria and ventricles serve to pump blood to the lungs to receive oxygen and then pump the oxygenated blood to the body. It does this an average of 70 times per minute. It receives deoxygenated blood from the body via veins. The veins deliver blood from tissues throughout the body, to the heart to be reoxygenated. Once the blood has been sent through the lungs, the oxygenated blood

Table 6-1

BODY STRUCTURES OF THE NERVOUS SYSTEM

Body Structure	Body Functions Reliant on This Structure	
Frontal lobe	Judgment Concept formation Metacognition Cognitive flexibility Insight Attention Awareness Sustained, selective, and divided attention Memory Temporal relationships Recognition Categorization Generalization Awareness of reality Logical/coherent thought	Appropriate thought content Execution of learned movement patterns Coping and behavioral regulation Emotional stability Motivation Impulse control Body image Self-concept Self-esteem Orientation Eye–hand/foot coordination Bilateral integration Crossing midline Fine and gross motor control Walking patterns
Temporal lobe	Concept formation Memory Discrimination of sensations (auditory) Recognition Categorization Generalization	Execution of learned movement patterns Coping and behavioral regulation Orientation Tolerance of ambient sounds Awareness of location and distance of sounds
Parietal lobe	Spatial relationships Discrimination of sensations (visual) Awareness of body position and space	Taste Touch Pain Thermal awareness
Occipital lobe	Detection/registration Modulation	Visual awareness of environment at various distances
Midbrain (Mesencephalon)	Discrimination of senses (auditory, visual) Execution of learned movement patterns Detection/registration Modulation Visual awareness at various distance Tolerance of ambient sounds	Awareness of location and distance of sounds Eye–hand/foot coordination Crossing midline Fine and gross motor control Oculomotor control Walking patterns

(continued)

Table 6-1

BODY STRUCTURES OF THE NERVOUS SYSTEM (CONTINUED)

Body Structure	Body Functions Reliant on This Structure	
Diencephalon	Judgment Concept formation Metacognition Cognitive flexibility Insight Attention Awareness Coping and behavioral regulation Body image Self-concept Self-esteem Execution of learned movement patterns Arousal, consciousness Orientation Sleep Discrimination of senses (auditory, tactile, visual, olfactory, gustatory, vestibular-proprioception) Multisensory processing	Modulation Integration of sensations from the body and environment Tolerance of ambient sounds Awareness of location and distance of sounds Sensation of securely moving against gravity Taste Smell Proprioception Touch Thermal awareness Eye–hand/foot coordination Bilateral integration Crossing midline Fine and gross motor control Walking patterns Blood pressure functions Endocrine system functions
Basal ganglia	Eye–hand/foot coordination Bilateral integration Crossing midline	Fine and gross motor control Walking patterns
Cerebellum	Eye–hand/foot coordination Crossing midline Fine and gross motor control Righting and supporting	Muscle tone Walking patterns Sensation of moving securely against gravity
Brainstem	Arousal Consciousness Sleep Modulation Visual awareness at various distances Sensations of securely moving against gravity Touch Pain	Oculomotor control Righting and supporting Eye–hand/foot coordination Bilateral integration Crossing the midline Fine and gross motor control Walking patterns Blood pressure functions Cardiovascular system functions

(continued)

Table 6-1

BODY STRUCTURES OF THE NERVOUS SYSTEM (CONTINUED)

Body Structure	*Body Functions Reliant on This Structure*	
Brainstem (continued)	Thermal awareness Tolerance of ambient sounds Awareness of location and distance of sounds	Respiratory functions Digestive system functions Urinary functions
Cranial nerves	Detection/registration Modulation Visual awareness of environment and various distances Awareness of location and distance of sounds Sensation of securely moving against gravity	Taste Smell Awareness of body position and space Touch Fine and gross motor coordination Oculomotor control Digestive system functions
Spinal cord	Awareness of body position and space Touch Pain Thermal awareness Muscle tone Asymmetrical and symmetrical tonic neck reflex Righting and supporting Eye–hand/foot coordination	Bilateral coordination Crossing midline Fine and gross motor control Walking patterns Blood pressure functions Heart rate Voice functions Digestive system functions Urinary functions Genital and reproductive functions
Spinal nerves	Awareness of body position and space Touch Pain Thermal awareness Muscle tone Asymmetrical and symmetrical tonic neck reflex Righting and supporting Eye–hand/foot coordination	Bilateral coordination Crossing midline Fine and gross motor control Walking patterns Blood pressure functions Heart rate Voice functions Digestive system functions Urinary functions Genital and reproductive functions
Meninges	Judgment Concept formation Metacognition Cognitive flexibility Insight Attention Awareness	Self-concept Self-esteem Orientation Detection/registration Modulation Integration of sensations from the body and environment

(continued)

Table 6-1

BODY STRUCTURES OF THE NERVOUS SYSTEM (CONTINUED)

Body Structure	Body Functions Reliant on This Structure	
Meninges (continued)	Sustained, selective, and divided attention Memory Discrimination of sensations Multisensory processing Sensory memory Spatial relationships Temporal relationships Recognition Categorization Generalization Awareness of reality Logical/coherent thought Appropriate thought content Execution of learned movement patterns Coping and behavioral regulation Emotional stability Motivation Impulse control Body image	Visual awareness of environment at various distances Tolerance of ambient sounds Awareness of location and distance of sounds Sensation of securely moving against gravity Awareness of body position and space Localizing pain Thermal awareness Muscle tone Asymmetrical tonic neck reflex Symmetrical tonic neck reflex Righting and supporting Eye–hand/foot coordination Bilateral integration Crossing midline Fine and gross motor control Oculomotor control Walking patterns
Sympathetic nervous system	Detection/registration Modulation Integration of sensations from body and environment	Visual awareness of environment at various distances Blood pressure functions Rate, rhythm, and depth of respiration Digestive system function
Parasympathetic nervous system	Detection/registration Modulation Integration of sensations from body and environment	Visual awareness of environment at various distances Blood pressure functions Rate, rhythm, and depth of respiration Digestive system function

Table 6-2

EYES, EARS, AND RELATED STRUCTURES

Body Structure	Body Functions Reliant on This Structure
Eyeball: Conjunctiva, cornea, iris, retina, lens, vitreous body	Detection/registration Modulation Integration of sensations from the body and environment Visual awareness at various distances Eye–hand/foot coordination
Structures around eye: Lacrimal gland, eyelid, eyebrow, external ocular muscles	Detection/registration Integration of sensations from the body and environment Visual awareness at various distances Eye–hand/foot coordination Oculomotor
Structure of external ear	Awareness of location and distance of sounds
Structure of middle ear: Tympanic membrane, eustachian canal, ossicles	Awareness of location and distance of sounds
Structures of inner ear: Cochlea, vestibular labyrinth, semicircular canals, internal auditory meatus	Awareness of location and distance of sounds Sensation of securely moving against gravity Awareness of body position Righting and supporting Walking patterns

Table 6-3

STRUCTURES INVOLVED IN VOICE AND SPEECH FUNCTIONS

Body Structure	Body Functions Reliant on This Structure
Structures of the nose: External nose, nasal septum, nasal fossae	Voice functions Fluency and rhythm Alternative vocalization
Structure of the mouth: Teeth, gums, hard palate, soft palate, tongue, lips	Voice functions Fluency and rhythm Alternative vocalization
Structure of pharynx: Nasal pharynx and oral pharynx	Voice functions Fluency and rhythm Alternative vocalization
Structure of larynx: Vocal folds	Voice functions Fluency and rhythm Alternative vocalization

Table 6-4

BODY STRUCTURES OF THE CARDIOVASCULAR SYSTEM

Body structure	Body functions reliant on this structure
Heart: Atria, ventricles	Level of arousal and consciousness
	Blood pressure functions
	Heart rate
	Physical endurance
	Stamina and fatigability
Arteries	Blood pressure functions
	Muscle endurance
	Physical endurance
	Stamina and fatigability
Veins	Blood pressure functions
	Muscle endurance
	Physical endurance
	Stamina and fatigability
Capillaries	Blood pressure functions
	Muscle endurance

is sent out to the tissues of the body through arteries (*Mosby's Dictionary*, 2006). Capillaries are a network of thin-walled blood vessels where oxygenated blood from the arteries is delivered to the body and then returned to the heart through veins. Capillaries exist throughout the body providing oxygen and other nutrients to tissue via the blood (Youngstrom, 2000) (See Table 6-4).

Immune System

The immune system functions to protect the body against infection and disease. The body protects itself through an elaborate system that includes the thymus, bone marrow, lymph tissues, lymph nodes, spleen, and lymph vessels (*Mosby's Dictionary*, 2006). The thymus is a lymph gland located around the sternum area and is the primary site for the creation of T cells. T cells originate in the bone marrow, but are sent to the thymus to mature, after which they travel to other lymph tissues in the body to fight off antigens or foreign substances (*Taber's Cyclopedic Medical Dictionary*, 2001). Lymph nodes are small kidney-shaped collections of tissue from which lymph fluid flows. Antibodies are produced in the lymph nodes and then travel to the blood via the lymph fluid. Lymph nodes are located throughout the body, either singly or in clusters along the lymphatic vessels

which run from the head, down the neck and into the arms, through the trunk and down the legs (*Taber's Cyclopedic Medical Dictionary*, 2001). The spleen is also essential to the immune system in that it creates lymphocytes and antibodies to help fight off invaders to the body. The spleen also works to remove cell debris, old or damaged cells, and cells that are coated with antibodies (*Taber's Cyclopedic Medical Dictionary*, 2001). It is located in the upper left quadrant of the abdomen, near the stomach (See Table 6-5).

Respiratory System

The respiratory system structures serve to bring oxygen into the body via the blood. This occurs by inhalation, which is controlled by movement of the intercostal muscles surrounding the rib cage, as well as the diaphragm. When the diaphragm contracts, it flattens itself downward, away from the lungs, creating pressure which allows the lungs to expand. When the lungs are allowed to expand, air is pulled in through the trachea, a tube made of cartilage that extends from the larynx down to two branches, one to each lung. Protecting and surrounding the lungs and heart is the thoracic cage, which consists of the 12 pairs of rib bones, the sternum, and the thoracic vertebrae that run up the back side of the cage. The thoracic cage moves along with inspiration and

Table 6-5

BODY STRUCTURES OF THE IMMUNE SYSTEM

Body Structure	Body Functions Reliant on This Structure
Lymphatic vessels	Joint range of motion Walking patterns Immunological system functions Protective functions of the skin Repair functions of the skin
Lymphatic nodes	Joint range of motion Walking patterns Protective functions of the skin Repair functions of the skin Immunological system functions
Thymus	Immunological system functions Protective functions of the skin Repair functions of the skin
Spleen	Immunological system functions Protective functions of the skin Repair functions of the skin
Bone marrow	Immunological system functions Protective functions of the skin Repair functions of the skin

expiration and provides the structure needed for negative and positive airway pressure that pulls air in and out with each contraction and relaxation of the diaphragm (See Table 6-6).

STRUCTURES RELATED TO THE DIGESTIVE, METABOLIC, AND ENDOCRINE SYSTEMS

The digestive, metabolic, and endocrine systems work together to effectively utilize food as an energy source. The digestive system begins its work as food enters the mouth and the salivary glands produce saliva to begin breaking down food particles. As food is swallowed, it travels down the esophagus to the stomach where the digestion process begins. Protein digestion begins in the stomach, but most absorption of food occurs in the small intestine. The stomach does absorb liquids, however. Food travels from the stomach to the small intestine where it is joined by bile from the liver and gallbladder and pancreatic juice from the pancreas. It is in the small intestine that essential nutrients and fluids are absorbed into the blood, which is then sent to the liver. The liver has multiple functions related to metabolizing food molecules to be utilized. The liver also detoxifies the blood stream by working to break down harmful substances, such as alcohol or drugs. Hemoglobin by-products are broken down and sent out into the feces to be eliminated. The liver also produces protein and clotting factors, as well as stores copper, iron, and vitamins B_{12}, A, D, E, and K (*Taber's Cyclopedic Medical Dictionary*, 2001). Endocrine glands excrete hormones directly into the blood stream. The pituitary, thyroid, parathyroid, and adrenal glands all contribute to metabolic activities (the utilization of food and water that is put into the body), growth, and sexual development and functions (See Table 6-7).

Table 6-6

BODY STRUCTURES OF THE RESPIRATORY SYSTEM

Body Structure	Body Functions Reliant on This Structure	
Trachea	Respiratory system functions Rate, rhythm, and depth of respiration Physical endurance Aerobic capacity	Stamina Fatigability Voice functions Alternative vocalization functions
Lungs: Bronchial tree, alveoli	Respiratory system functions Rate, rhythm, and depth of respiration Physical endurance Aerobic capacity	Stamina Fatigability Voice functions Alternative vocalization functions
Thoracic cage	Respiratory system functions Rate, rhythm, and depth of respiration Physical endurance Aerobic capacity	Stamina Fatigability Voice functions Alternative vocalization functions
Muscles of respiration: Intercostal muscles, diaphragm	Respiratory system functions Rate, rhythm, and depth of respiration Physical endurance Aerobic capacity	Stamina Fatigability Voice functions Alternative vocalization functions

Table 6-7

STRUCTURES OF THE DIGESTIVE, METABOLIC, AND ENDOCRINE SYSTEMS

Body Structure	Body Functions Reliant on This Structure	
Salivary glands	Association of taste	Digestive system functions
Esophagus	Digestive system functions	
Stomach	Digestive system functions	Metabolic system
Intestines: Small and large	Digestive system functions	Metabolic system
Pancreas	Digestive system functions	Metabolic system
Liver	Digestive system functions Immunological system functions	Metabolic system Endocrine system
Gallbladder and ducts	Digestive system functions	Metabolic system
Endocrine glands: Pituitary, thyroid, parathyroid, adrenal	Digestive system functions Metabolic system functions Endocrine system functions	Genital and reproductive functions Hair and nail functions Emotional stability Appetite

Table 6-8

STRUCTURES OF THE GENITOURINARY AND REPRODUCTIVE SYSTEMS

Body Structure	Body Functions Reliant on This Structure
Urinary system: Kidneys, ureters, bladder, urethra	Urinary functions
Structure of pelvic floor	Reproductive functions Walking patterns
Structure of reproductive system: Ovaries, uterus, breast and nipple, vagina and external genitalia, testes, penis, prostate	Reproductive functions

STRUCTURES RELATED TO THE GENITOURINARY AND REPRODUCTIVE SYSTEMS

The structures of the genitourinary system relate to all structures which allow for urination and reproduction. In men, many of the structures are shared for urination and for reproduction; in women, most of the structures are separate. The urinary system is comprised of the kidneys, which serve to filter the blood and eliminate wastes through the urine. The urine that is created in the kidneys is sent to the bladder via the ureter, which is a tube that runs from each kidney into the bladder. From the bladder, the urine passes through the urethra out of the body. The pelvic floor is comprised of muscles and ligaments that hold the pelvic organs, which include the muscles required for urination, as well as those needed to support the reproductive organs. A failure in the functioning of the pelvic floor is one of the leading causes of urinary incontinence (*Mosby's Dictionary*, 2006). Structures of the female reproductive system include the ovaries, uterus, breast, nipple, and external genitalia; the male reproductive system includes the testes, penis, and prostate. The male relies on the structures of the penis and prostrate for urination as well (See Table 6-8).

STRUCTURES RELATED TO MOVEMENT

Of all of the body structure categories, this has the greatest number of related structures involved. When analyzing an activity that requires movement, it will be important to identify the specific body structures required for the task. For this reason, the ICF details very specific muscular and joint structures of all areas of the body. Determining which of these structures is needed for an activity will require an examination of each of the steps and specific movements required of each body part (See Table 6-9).

SKIN AND RELATED STRUCTURES

The structures related to skin and hair are part of many grooming and bathing activities such as washing hair and trimming nails. Thus, these body structures would be required of those occupations. Without hair, the task of washing one's hair becomes unneeded. Thus, for this body structure category, it easier to think of what occupations or activities hair, skin, and nails are required for, instead of thinking of what body functions are reliant on these structures (See Table 6-10).

Table 6-9

BODY STRUCTURES RELATED TO MOVEMENT

Body Structure	Body Functions Reliant on This Structure	
Bones of cranium	None	
Bones of face	Digestive system functions	
Bones of neck region	Asymmetrical tonic neck reflex Symmetrical tonic reflex	
Joints of head and neck	Digestive system functions Joint range of motion (head and neck)	Asymmetrical tonic neck reflex Symmetrical tonic reflex Righting and supporting reflex
Bones of shoulder region	Asymmetrical tonic neck reflex Symmetrical tonic reflex Righting and supporting reflex	
Joints of shoulder region	Joint range of motion (shoulder) Postural alignment (shoulder) Asymmetrical tonic neck reflex	Symmetrical tonic reflex Righting and supporting reflex
Muscles of shoulder region	Strength (shoulder) Endurance Asymmetrical tonic neck reflex	Symmetrical tonic reflex Righting and supporting reflex
Bones of upper arm	Asymmetrical tonic neck reflex Symmetrical tonic reflex Righting and supporting reflex	
Elbow joint	Joint range of motion (elbow) Postural alignment Asymmetrical tonic neck reflex	Symmetrical tonic reflex Righting and supporting reflex
Muscles of upper arm	Strength Symmetrical tonic reflex	Asymmetrical tonic neck reflex Righting and supporting reflex
Ligaments and fascia of upper arm	Joint range of motion (upper arm)	
Bones of forearm	Asymmetrical tonic neck reflex Righting and supporting reflex	Symmetrical tonic reflex
Wrist joint	Joint range of motion (wrist) Righting and supporting	Postural alignment
Muscles of forearm	Strength	Righting and supporting
Ligaments and fascia of forearm	Joint range of motion (forearm)	

(continued)

Table 6-9

BODY STRUCTURES RELATED TO MOVEMENT (CONTINUED)

Body Structure	Body Functions Reliant on This Structure	
Bones of hand	Righting and supporting	
Joints of hand and fingers	Joint range of motion Righting and supporting	Postural alignment
Muscles of hand	Righting and supporting	
Ligaments and fascia of hand	Joint range of motion	
Bones of pelvic region	Righting and supporting	
Joints of pelvic region	Joint range of motion Righting and supporting	Postural alignment
Muscles of pelvic region	Righting and supporting	
Ligaments and fascia of pelvic region	Joint range of motion Righting and supporting	Postural alignment
Bones of thigh	Righting and supporting	
Hip joint	Joint range of motion Righting and supporting	Postural alignment
Muscles of thigh	Righting and supporting	
Ligaments and fascia of thigh	Joint range of motion Righting and supporting	Postural alignment
Bones of lower leg	Righting and supporting	
Knee joint	Joint range of motion	Postural alignment
Muscles of lower leg	Righting and supporting	
Ligaments and fascia of lower leg	Joint range of motion Righting and supporting	Postural alignment
Bones of ankle and foot	Righting and supporting	
Ankle, foot, and toe joints	Joint range of motion Righting and supporting	Postural alignment
Muscle of ankle and foot	Righting and supporting	
Ligaments and fascia of ankle and foot	Joint range of motion Righting and supporting	Postural alignment
Cervical vertebral column	Joint range of motion	Postural alignment
Lumbar vertebral column	Joint range of motion	Postural alignment
Sacral vertebral column	Joint range of motion	Postural alignment
Coccyx	Joint range of motion	Postural alignment
Muscles of trunk	Righting and supporting	
Ligaments and fascia of trunk	Joint range of motion	

Table 6-10

SKIN AND RELATED STRUCTURES

Body Structure	Body Functions Reliant on This Structure
Areas of skin: Head, neck, shoulder, upper extremity, pelvic region, lower extremities, trunk and back	Joint mobility Touch functions Pain Temperature and pressure Protective functions of the skin Repair functions of the skin
Structure of skin glands: Sweat and sebaceous	Protective functions of the skin Repair functions of the skin
Structure of nails: Fingernails, toenails	Hair and nail functions
Structure of hair	Hair and nail functions

CONCLUSION

Body structures are those physical aspects of organs, limbs, and structures of each organ that support body functioning. Structures work together to keep the human body healthy and allow for participation in daily activities. The extent to which each body structure is challenged relies on the demands of the activities (the steps, space, objects, and social demands) and is linked to the body functions utilized. As OT practitioners, it is important to recognize the importance of each of the body systems and how each one can influence performance of activities. The body systems work collaboratively and are often not solely responsible for a single function. For example, many of our mental functions not only rely on the structures on the nervous system but also rely on the cardiovascular system's ability to deliver oxygen-rich blood to the brain in order to function. While this chapter offers a brief introduction to the primary functions of each body system, understand that the body is much more complex and further investigation into a specific system is warranted for specialization.

QUESTIONS

1. Washing hair in the shower challenges which body structures (beyond what is required to sustain life)?

2. Why is it necessary to know which body structures are required of an activity?

3. How do you determine which body structures are necessary for an activity?

4. What are the structures of the nervous system? What are at least 10 body functions the nervous system structures support?

5. What body functions do the lymph structures support?

6. Voice functions are supported by which body structures?

ACTIVITY

1. Body structure charades: Each of the following body structures will be written on a piece of paper and placed in a hat or bowl:
   - Frontal lobe
   - Temporal lobe
   - Parietal lobe
   - Occipital lobe
   - Eyeball: Conjunctiva, cornea, iris, retina, lens, vitreous body
   - Structures around eye: Lacrimal gland, eyelid, eyebrow, external ocular muscles
   - Structure of external ear

- Structure of middle ear: Tympanic membrane, eustachian canal, ossicles
- Structures of inner ear: Cochlea, vestibular labyrinth, semicircular canals, internal auditory meatus
- Structures of the nose: External nose, nasal septum, nasal fossae
- Structure of the mouth: Teeth, gums, hard palate, soft palate, tongue, lips
- Structure of pharynx: Nasal pharynx and oral pharynx
- Structure of larynx: Vocal folds
- Salivary glands
- Esophagus
- Stomach
- Urinary system: Kidneys, ureters, bladder, urethra
- Structure of reproductive system: Ovaries, uterus, breast and nipple, vagina and external genitalia, testes, penis, prostate
- Bones of cranium
- Bones of face
- Bones of neck region
- Joints of head and neck
- Bones of shoulder region
- Joints of shoulder region
- Muscles of shoulder region
- Bones of upper arm
- Elbow joint
- Muscles of upper arm
- Ligaments and fascia of upper arm
- Bones of forearm
- Wrist joint
- Muscles of forearm
- Ligaments and fascia of forearm
- Bones of hand
- Joints of hand and fingers
- Muscles of hand
- Bones of pelvic region
- Joints of pelvic region
- Muscles of pelvic region
- Bones of thigh
- Hip joint
- Muscles of thigh
- Bones of lower leg
- Knee joint
- Muscles of lower leg
- Bones of ankle and foot
- Ankle, foot and toe joints
- Muscle of ankle and foot
- Cervical vertebral column
- Lumbar vertebral column
- Muscles of trunk
- Areas of skin: Head, neck, shoulder, upper extremity, pelvic region, lower extremities, trunk, and back
- Structure of skin glands: Sweat and sebaceous
- Structure of nails: Fingernails, toenails
- Structure of hair

Each student will draw one of the body structures and then act out or pantomime an activity in which the body structure is required. The class is to guess which body structure the activity is utilizing.

2. An adaptation of the activity above: Each student draws a body structure from the hat or bowl. Each person is given one minute to write down as many activities that he or she can think of that require that body structure. At the one minute mark, the students are to pass it to the person next to them (each student gets his or her neighbor's sheet) and are given one minute to think of other activities which have not already been listed.

REFERENCES

American Occupational Therapy Association. (2008). Occupational therapy practice framework: Domain and process (2nd ed.). *American Journal of Occupational Therapy, 62*(6), 609–639.

Blessing, W. (2002). Functions Regulated in the Brain Stem. In V. Ramachandran (Ed.) *Encyclopedia of the human brain.* San Francisco, CA: Elsevier Science & Technology.

Butler, A. (2002). Cranial Nerves. In V. Ramachandran (Ed.), *Encyclopedia of the human brain.* San Francisco, CA: Elsevier Science & Technology.

Craighead, E., & Nemeroff, C. (Eds.)(2004). Brain. In *The concise Corsini encyclopedia of psychology and behavioral ccience.* Indianapolis, IN: John Wiley & Sons, Inc.

Crosson, B., Maron, L., Moore, A. & Grande, L. (2002). Basal Ganglia. In V. Ramachandran (Ed.) *Encyclopedia of the human brain.* San Francisco, CA: Elsevier Science & Technology.

Filley, C. (2002). Neuroanatomy. In V. Ramachandran (Ed.) *Encyclopedia of the human brain.* San Francisco, CA: Elsevier Science & Technology.

Molinari, M. (2002). Cerebellum. In V. Ramachandran (Ed.), *Encyclopedia of the human brain.* San Francisco, CA: Elsevier Science & Technology.

Mosby's dictionary of medicine , nursing & health professions. (2006). St. Louis, MO: Author.

Taber's cyclopedic medical dictionary. (2001). Philadelphia, PA: F.A. Davis Company.

Walker, R., & Parker, S. (2009). *The human body book: An illustrated guide to its structure, function and disorders.* London, UK: Dorling Kindersley

World Health Organization. (2001). *International classification of functioning, disability, and health.* Geneva, Switzerland: Author.

Youngstrom, R. (2000). *The royal society of medicine health encyclopedia.* London, UK: Bloomsbury Publishing.

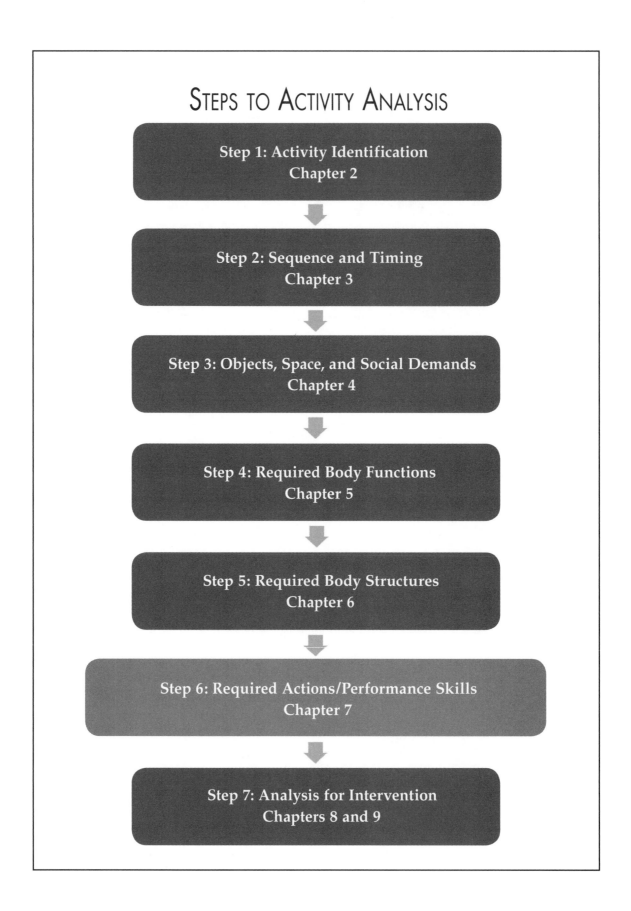

7

REQUIRED ACTIONS / PERFORMANCE SKILLS

OBJECTIVES

1. Define what performance skills are and how they are different from body functions.

2. Understand what can influence performance skills using perspectives from frames of reference and ecological models.

3. Distinguish how to determine the skill level required of an activity.

4. Identify the elements of motor and praxis skills and the body functions influencing these skills.

5. Define the elements of sensory perceptual skills and the body functions influencing these skills.

6. Identify the different aspects of emotional regulation skills and the body functions that influence these skills.

7. Define the aspects of cognitive skills and the body functions that influence these skills.

8. Identify the different aspects of communication and social skills and the body functions influencing these skills.

The next step in the activity analysis process is determining the required actions or performance skills. Performance skills are defined as "observable, concrete, goal-directed actions" that are used to perform meaningful tasks (American Occupational Therapy Association [AOTA], 2008, p. 639). Performance skills are therefore abilities that are demonstrated through actions and have the potential to be learned and improved over time. Performance skills are assessed as they are performed by a client as they perform an activity or the skill level needed is determined prior to execution of the activity, as conducted in an activity analysis. Determining the skills required of an activity requires examination of the steps used to carry out the activity as well as the required body functions, objects, environment, and social demands. It is for this reason that determining the performance skills is not conducted earlier in the activity analysis process. Each action and performance skill is supported by body functions and structures. Identifying these aspects of the activity demands first provides a link to understanding the level of performance skill required in each area.

Ecological models and theories are foundational to occupational therapy's understanding of performance. The three models used in occupational therapy (OT) practice are the Ecology of Human Performance model, The Person Environment Occupational Performance model, and the Person Environment Occupation (PEO) model. All three of these models contend that ability to perform in an occupation is influenced not only by the aspects of the person (the body functions, beliefs, values) but also by aspects of the occupation (the objects and properties, social demands, sequence and timing) and the environment (the space demands and physical context). Using this frame in which to understand performance, the skill level needed to perform an activity is measured by not only the body functions utilized but the activity and the environment it is performed in. As a change in the environment occurs, the skill level may increase or decrease. The same is true for changes in aspects of the occupation. For example,

Thomas, H. *Occupation-Based Activity Analysis* (pp. 125-138).
© 2012 SLACK Incorporated

Figure 7-1. The PEO model: influence of the person, environment, and occupation on performance.

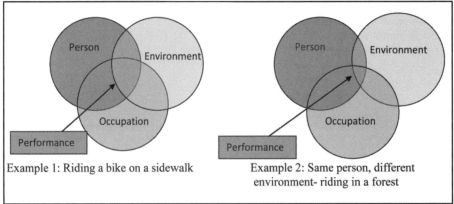

Example 1: Riding a bike on a sidewalk   Example 2: Same person, different environment- riding in a forest

the skill level needed to ride a bike increases when the surface and environment become more complex, such as riding through a forest. See Figure 7-1 for an illustration of how a change in one aspect can influence performance.

The area in the center of the diagram where all three circles overlap indicates the performance of the occupation being engaged in. As one of the areas moves or changes, such as in Example 2 where the environment changes, performance shrinks. This demonstrates the view that performance is influenced not only by skill and body functions with the person but by the activity itself and the contexts in which it is performed.

The *Occupational Therapy Practice Framework, 2nd Edition* (*Framework*) has delineated five broad areas of performance skill: motor and praxis, sensory–perceptual, emotional regulation, cognitive, and communication/social skills (AOTA, 2008). The level of skill identified should be that which "would be required by any performer to carry out the activity" (AOTA, 2008, p. 638). For example, a moderate amount of motor and praxis skill is required to shampoo hair while in the shower. The person must maneuver his or her body and head under the water, reach for the shampoo bottle, open the bottle, squeeze the right amount into the opposite hand, set the bottle down, and then massage the shampoo into the hair. This is the skill level required for most people to complete the activity. For many activities, interactions of different performance skills influence successful engagement in the activity. Social interaction skills may be influenced by motor and praxis ability or communication and social skills may be impacted by emotional regulation skills. For example, if a person is giving a speech, the person's emotional regulation skills (ability to stay calm with so many people watching her) will influence her communication skills.

To understand how much each performance skill influences successful engagement in the activity, examine each category of performance skill individually. For each area, is a low, medium, or

high skill level required? Think about all of the steps required to complete the activity. Look back at your analysis of the body functions required for the activity; this can direct you toward identifying the performance skills needed. For example, decorating a cake requires a high level of fine and gross motor coordination, eye–hand coordination, and strength in the hands; thus, motor and praxis skills are in high demand. However, it requires low emotional regulation skill level, as there are few actions required that challenge the person to control their expression of feelings.

Also think about the environment in which the activity takes place. The surface and space may influence the required skill. For example, a low level of motor and praxis skill is needed to go down a beginner ski slope versus the skill level needed for an expert slope. The social demands of the activity may also have an impact of the skill level required. Be sure to have a good understanding of the objects and properties utilized as well, as some objects may be more difficult to use than others. All of this will make more sense as we delve into defining each performance skill area.

MOTOR AND PRAXIS SKILLS

The *Framework* combines motor and praxis together, as they are inter-related and dependent on each other for engagement in activities. Motor skills are required in order to move and interact with the environment and objects in it. In order to move in the needed manner, the movements must be planned out and executed in a sequential fashion. *Praxis* is the ability to carry out sequential movements, with the correct timing and transitions between one movement and another. It is often called *motor planning* as it relates to planning and executing functional movements. Humans develop praxis skills as infants, learning how to control movement, transitioning from a baby who is able to move randomly and nonpurposefully to

Table 7-1

MOTOR AND PRAXIS SKILLS: BODY FUNCTIONS UTILIZED

- Execution of learned movement patterns
- Level of arousal
- Level of consciousness
- Sensation of securely moving against gravity
- Awareness of body position and pace
- Joint range of motion
- Joint postural alignment
- Strength
- Degree of muscle tone
- Muscle endurance
- Stretch, ATNR, and STNR reflexes

- Righting and supporting
- Eye–hand/foot coordination
- Bilateral integration
- Crossing midline
- Fine and gross motor control
- Oculomotor control
- Walking patterns
- Blood pressure functions
- Heart rate
- Respiratory rate, rhythm, and depth

being able to reach for objects or turn the head toward something of interest. Gaining praxis ability means that movements become more natural, in that we do not need to think about what we need to do in order to move. Think about when you brush your teeth in the morning. Do you think about how you are going to move your arm to reach for the toothbrush? Unless you are very sleepy, you do not have to think about it, and your arm automatically moves in a controlled fashion to reach forward and grasp the handle.

The level of motor and praxis skills required for an activity goes up as the objects, space, and social demands go up. If the objects being used become more difficult to maneuver (for example, using small buttons versus big buttons), then the challenge for fine finger movements will go up. If the physical environment provides greater challenges, then the requirements for greater control over movements will increase. The social expectations and demands may also influence the skill level required of an activity. For example, if writing a note to yourself, the motor/praxis skill needed is low, as there is no social expectation for legibility. However, if writing the address on an envelope that will be going in the mail, there is a moderate level of motor/praxis skill required as it must be read by the workers in the post office.

The *Framework* utilizes literature from several different sources to clarify the meaning of motor and praxis skills:

+ Motor:
  - "Actions or behaviors a client uses to move and physically interact with tasks, objects, contexts, and environments."

  - "Includes planning, sequencing, and executing new and novel movements" (AOTA, 2008, p. 640).

+ Praxis:
  - "Skilled purposeful movements."
  - "Ability to carry out sequential motor acts as part of an overall plan rather than individual acts."
  - "Ability to carry out learned motor activity, including following through on a verbal command, visual-spatial construction, ocular and oral-motor skills, imitation of a person or an object, and sequencing actions."
  - "Organization of temporal sequences of actions within the spatial context which form meaningful occupations" (AOTA, 2008, p. 640).

Obtaining motor and praxis skills requires the utilization of several body functions, many of which work in conjunction with each other to produce purposeful movement. Of course, simply having a body function does not imply skill level or ability (AOTA, 2008). Motor and praxis skills are actions that are observable and utilize a variety of body functions. Table 7-1 is a list of the possible body functions that underlie motor/praxis skills.

Table 7-2 gives examples of activities and the motor and praxis skill level required.

Table 7-2

EXAMPLE OF ANALYSIS OF REQUIRED MOTOR/PRAXIS SKILLS

Activity/Task	Low	Mod	High	Examples of Motor/Praxis Actions
Bowling for fun		X		Bending down to pick up the ball Grasping the ball with both hands Coordinating fingers to insert into holes Pacing movements to swing ball toward pins Aligning body and ball toward pins Adjusting body posture in response to movement of the ball
Washing a window		X		Grasping the bottle of cleaner Aligning the body and arm toward the window Coordinating the fingers to contract with the appropriate force to spray cleaner Calibrating the amount of force needed to hold the towel against the glass without breaking it Reaching all areas of the window Adjusting posture and body position in response to reaching to all areas of the window
Threading a needle		X		Coordinating the use of both hands together Grasping the needle and thread Maintaining stable body and arms while moving fingers Coordinating small movements in response to visual and tactile information
Riding the bus	X			Coordinating trunk and lower body to climb stairs into bus Manipulating change to pay fare Anticipating and adjusting posture and body position as the bus moves
Reading a book	X			Grasping book with one or both hands Manipulating pages to flip a single page Coordinating eyes to scan the page

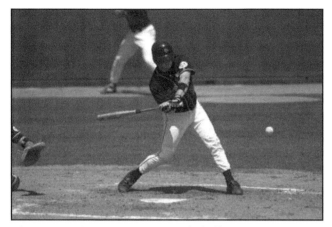

Figure 7-2. Sensory-perceptual skills are required to swing the bat at the ball.

SENSORY-PERCEPTUAL SKILLS

Understanding and perceiving the sensory information we receive from our surroundings is a skill. Actions we take in response to the environment require detecting and identifying the sensory information correctly, interpreting what the sensation means, and associating that sensation with a past event or storing it in memory for associating in the future. For example, as a small child, we may not understand what the sound of screeching car tires means. As we get older, we begin to have experiences that teach us to discriminate between the sound of tires making noise because the vehicle is taking off quickly and the noise it makes when stopping very quickly. We begin to associate each sound, the pitch, and intensity of each sound with what we believe to be occurring (such as a car accident or a car skidding to miss a cat or dog in the street). If we were walking across the street and suddenly heard the sound of screeching tires, our ability to identify and respond to the sound leads us to action, such as moving away from the direction of the sound.

Sensory perceptual skills are also used to differentiate between tastes, smells, and textures. It is sensory perceptual skills that allow us to stick our hand in our pockets or purses and pull out the small item we are looking for without looking at it; we are able to identify objects simply by touch. Visual perceptual skills are what allow us to identify objects, discriminating based on size, shape, and color. It is also what allows us to perceive depth and texture by sight. Proprioceptive skills are the ability to perceive the body's position in space and the movement of body parts. As this skill improves, we are able to move with greater precision and control and able to move our body parts without the use of vision to know where we are moving. For example, when a person learns to play baseball, he uses his proprioceptive skills to determine where he is holding the bat and what angle to swing it at, without looking at the bat or his arms (Figure 7-2).

Table 7-3 is a list of the possible body functions that underlie sensory-perceptive skills. Table 7-4 gives examples of activities and the sensory-perceptual skill level required.

EMOTIONAL REGULATION SKILLS

Emotions are feelings or a psychological or mental response to internal or external events (*Mosby's Dictionary*, 2006). How we react or express these feelings when engaged in an activity requires regulation. Emotional regulation is a person's ability to identify his or her emotions and manage them effectively and appropriately for the activity or setting. The level of emotional regulation required of an activity is very dependent on the social demands of the activity. It is also reliant on the intrinsic rewards or outcomes of the activity. For example, flying a kite can cause great laughter and happiness, an outcome difficult to predict based on the activity demands.

Emotions can range from the positive, such as love, happiness, and excitement, to the negative, such as hatred, sorrow, frustration, and fear (this is a very limited list of the range of emotions that humans can feel). In conducting an activity analysis, it is not necessary to identify what emotions may be evoked during the activity but how much the person will be challenged to regulate or manage the expression of their emotions. For example, if playing a game of chess, the loser must not express his or her unhappiness about losing by throwing objects or punching out the winner. Behaviors related to emotional expression may also be required for activities where there are no other people around, but it is required in order to allow continuation of the activity. For example, while learning how to play the piano (Figure 7-3), Charlotte has difficulty hitting the right keys. If she allows herself to get too frustrated, she might quit trying to play. Managing one's emotions allows us to address the difficulties and triumphs in life and continue on.

Table 7-3

SENSORY-PERCEPTUAL SKILLS: BODY FUNCTIONS UTILIZED

- Discrimination of senses (auditory, tactile, visual, olfactory, gustatory, vestibular-proprioception)
- Multisensory processing
- Sensory memory
- Spatial relationships
- Temporal relationships
- Recognition
- Categorization
- Generalization
- Detection/registration
- Modulation
- Integration of sensations for the body and environment

- Visual awareness of environment at various distances
- Tolerance of ambient sounds
- Awareness of location and distance of sounds
- Sensation of securely moving against gravity
- Association of taste
- Association of smell
- Awareness of body position and space
- Comfort with the feeling of being touched
- Localizing pain
- Thermal awareness

Table 7-4

EXAMPLES OF ANALYSIS OF REQUIRED SENSORY-PERCEPTUAL SKILLS

Activity/task	Low	Mod	High	Examples of sensory processing actions
Bowling for fun		X		Visually determine where the pins are and how far away Positioning the body toward the pins and swinging arm behind and in front of body Maintaining balance based on vestibular input from position changes
Washing a window		X		Visually detecting where the window is, where the cleaner is sprayed, and what still needs to be cleaned Determining level of pressure being applied to window

(continued)

Table 7-4

EXAMPLES OF ANALYSIS OF REQUIRED SENSORY-PERCEPTUAL SKILLS (CONTINUED)

Activity/Task	Low	Mod	High	Examples of Sensory Processing Actions
Threading a needle		X		Visually attending to and focusing on thread and small hole on needle Locating and maintaining location of thread in fingers
Riding the bus		X		Visually identifying the correct bus and destination Utilizing vestibular information as bus moves to maintain balance Hearing the bus driver announce locations along route
Reading a book	X			Discriminating between shapes and colors to discern between letters and characters Feeling for one page with fingertips in order to turn the page

Figure 7-3. Learning a new activity involves emotional regulation.

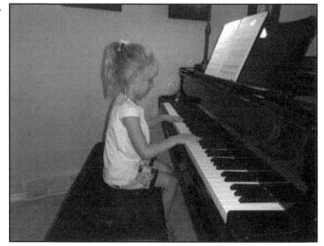

Table 7-5

EMOTIONAL REGULATION SKILLS: BODY FUNCTIONS UTILIZED

- Appropriate thought content
- Coping
- Behavioral regulation
- Body image
- Self-concept

- Self-esteem
- Emotional stability
- Motivation
- Impulse control
- Appetite

Table 7-5 is a list of the possible body functions that underlie emotional regulation skills. Table 7-6 gives examples of activities and the emotional regulation skill level required.

COGNITIVE SKILLS

Cognitive skills are what allow us to plan and manage our way through the steps of an activity and respond to changes in the environment as they occur. It is what allows us to select the appropriate objects and environment for the activity, as well as the appropriate time to conduct the activity. Cognitive ability is what allows us to identify problems and identify solutions to the problems. Cognitive skills also allow us to be creative and to multitask. All thinking-related tasks require cognitive skills that utilize a variety of the mental functions (Table 7-7). In order to actively participate in an occupation, the person must utilize some level of cognitive skill. Automatic or reflexive movements that are out of the control of the person performing them are considered void of requiring cognitive skills. For example, a person who flinches when a ball is thrown at him or her may be reacting automatically out of self-protection. Cognitive skill would be required if the person was to move away from the ball. In order to identify the skill level required for an activity, think about the complexity of the activity. Does it require sequencing, problem solving, organization, judgment, creativity, or multitasking? Are there multiple areas of cognition challenged and to what extent (basic knowledge or low challenge, or highly challenging)?

Table 7-7 is a list of the possible body functions that underlie cognitive skills. Table 7-8 gives examples of activities and the cognitive skill level required.

COMMUNICATION AND SOCIAL SKILLS

Communication occurs not only through speech but through gestures, facial expressions, written word, and creative arts. Communicating our needs and thoughts effectively is a skill that is gained over time. We communicate with others in order to have our needs met and to be understood. On a daily basis, we are communicating with others either directly or indirectly, such as in writing a paper or text messaging. Choosing the right words and timing of the words, sentences, and phrases are skills that can be sharpened over time.

The behaviors we exhibit when around and interacting with others are part of our social skills. How we act and behave when around others is part of what we are communicating to others about ourselves. Maintaining the appropriate physical space between the listener and speaker is a social skill. Initiating appropriate conversation, taking turns, and responding appropriately to a speaker are also social skills. Think of someone you may have met in which the interaction felt awkward or you felt that he or she had poor social skills. What behaviors did this person demonstrate that made you feel uncomfortable? Was his or her choice of topic inappropriate? Did he or she make rude bodily noises during conversation? Did this person use foul language? Perhaps he or she looked away and was distracted by the environment while you talked. All of these are examples of how the lack of social skills can detract from the effectiveness of communication.

The social skills required of an activity are very much reliant on the social demands for that particular activity. For example, the social demands, and thus the social skills, needed for bowling with friends for fun would be very different from those needed for

Table 7-6

EXAMPLES OF ANALYSIS OF REQUIRED EMOTIONAL REGULATION SKILLS

Activity/Task	Low	Mod	High	Examples of Emotional Regulation Actions
Bowling for fun	X			Controlling emotional display of disappointment or frustration Responding to the achievements or challenges of others appropriately
Washing a window	X			Persisting in the task despite difficulties
Threading a needle	X			Persisting in the task despite difficulties
Riding the bus		X		Display emotions appropriately around strangers Control display of anger or frustration if bus is late or unexpected events occur
Reading a book	X			Responding emotionally to what is being read

> **Table 7-7**
>
> ## Cognitive Skills: Body Functions Utilized
>
> - Judgment
> - Concept formation
> - Metacognition
> - Cognitive flexibility
> - Insight
> - Attention
> - Awareness
> - Sustained, selective, and divided attention
> - Short-term memory
> - Long-term memory
> - Working memory
>
> - Recognition
> - Categorization
> - Generalization
> - Awareness of reality
> - Logical/coherent thought
> - Appropriate thought content
> - Execution of learned movement patterns
> - Coping
> - Orientation to person, place, time, self, and others

bowling in a tournament. Thus, the language, use of physical space, touching, body language, turn-taking, and personal acknowledgments used during conversations can vary widely according to the setting and social demands. It is not uncommon for a person to use one set of social skills in one setting and quite a different set while in another (Figure 7-4). Do you communicate the same way while at school as you do at home with friends or family?

Communication and social skills go beyond the face-to-face and in-person interactions. Social skills are also utilized when on the telephone and when conducting online communications. The use of certain abbreviations (e.g., LOL for "laugh out loud") has become an acceptable term to use when communicating using text messaging, instant messaging, or e-mail. Thus, it is important to remember that communication and social skills are utilized in a variety of settings, including virtual environments.

Because communicating occurs via multiple avenues, not just through speech, there are many body functions that underlie and support the ability to communicate and demonstrate social skills. Mental functions are utilized during all methods of communication while the neuromusculoskeletal and movement-related functions are utilized when some type of movement is required. The respiratory system and voice and speech functions are utilized for communication that is verbally produced. See Table 7-9 for a list of all body functions that support communication and social skills. Table 7-10 gives

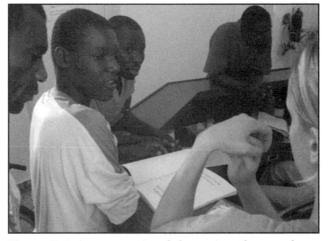

Figure 7-4. An occupational therapy student teaches Haitians medical information using body language.

examples of activities and the communication and social skill level required.

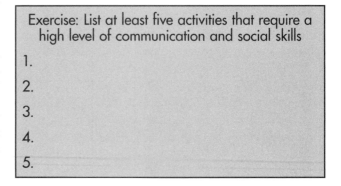

> Exercise: List at least five activities that require a high level of communication and social skills
>
> 1.
> 2.
> 3.
> 4.
> 5.

Table 7-8

EXAMPLES OF ANALYSIS OF REQUIRED COGNITIVE SKILLS

Activity/Task	Low	Mod	High	Examples of Cognitive Actions
Bowling for fun 		X		Choosing the correct ball Problem solving how to hit all of the pins Determining the winning score Following the rules of the game
Washing a window 	X			Selecting the correct objects needed Sequencing the steps in correct order
Threading a needle 	X			Sequencing the steps needed Problem solving how to get the thread through the small hole
Riding the bus 	X			Determining the correct amount to pay for the fare Judging when to stand to exit the bus at the correct stop Selecting the correct bus route and times to arrive at the desired location

Reading a book
 	
	X	X	X	Depending on the type of book:
				    Interpreting what is being read
				    Understanding what is being read

Table 7-9

COMMUNICATION AND SOCIAL SKILLS: BODY FUNCTIONS UTILIZED

- Judgment
- Concept formation
- Cognitive flexibility
- Insight
- Attention
- Awareness
- Sustained, selective, and divided attention
- Short-term memory
- Long-term memory
- Working memory
- Recognition
- Awareness of reality
- Logical/coherent thought
- Appropriate thought content
- Execution of learned movement patterns
- Orientation to person, place, time, self, and others
- Behavioral regulation
- Self-concept
- Self-esteem
- Emotional stability
- Motivation
- Impulse control
- Discrimination of senses (auditory, tactile, visual, vestibular-proprioception)
- Multisensory processing

- Sensory memory
- Spatial relationships
- Temporal relationships
- Modulation
- Integration of sensations for the body and environment
- Visual awareness of environment at various distances
- Tolerance of ambient sounds
- Awareness of location and distance of sounds
- Sensation of securely moving against gravity
- Awareness of body position and space
- Comfort with the feeling of being touched
- Joint range of motion
- Strength
- Righting and supporting
- Eye–hand/foot coordination
- Bilateral integration
- Crossing midline
- Fine and gross motor control
- Oculomotor control
- Respiratory rate, rhythm, and depth
- Voice functions
- Fluency and rhythm
- Alternative vocalization functions

CONCLUSION

Performance skills are observable actions that people demonstrate while engaged in an activity or occupation. As OT practitioners, we evaluate and assess this performance in our clients on a daily basis. We observe their performance looking for ways in which they may improve. By having an understanding of the level of skill required for an activity, we have a foundation by which to better understand how this performance may be changed. Perhaps it is the environment or the occupation that influences performance. In this chapter, we looked at performance skills not from the perspective of evaluating a client's skill level but by analyzing what amount of skill is required for an activity. Being able to look at occupations and activities from both perspectives allow clinicians to better understand how they can support greater participation.

QUESTIONS

1. How are performance skills different from body functions?

2. How do we determine how much skill is needed for an activity?

Table 7-10

EXAMPLES OF ANALYSIS OF REQUIRED COMMUNICATION AND SOCIAL SKILLS

Activity/Task	Low	Mod	High	Examples of Communication and Social Processing Actions
Bowling for fun		X		Gesturing to someone when he or she does well Taking turns when communicating
Washing a window				None
Threading a needle				None
Riding the bus	X			Asking the bus driver questions about the route Maintaining appropriate physical space when communicating to strangers
Reading a book				None

3. What external factors can influence the skill level of our clients?

4. How do OT practitioners use performance skills in practice?

5. Name one activity that requires high levels of all performance skills.

ACTIVITY

Identify the skills required of washing hair in the shower, indicating the level of skill required, giving examples of how each skill is used in the activity. See Appendix A for full form.

Skill	None	Low	Mod	High	Examples of how the skill is used
Motor/ praxis					
Sensory (perceptual)					
Emotional regulation					
Cognitive					
Communi- cation/social					

REFERENCES

American Occupational Therapy Association. (2008). Occupational therapy practice framework: Domain and process (2nd ed.). *American Journal of Occupational Therapy, 62,* 625–683.

Mosby's dictionary of medicine, nursing & health professions. (2006) St. Louis, MO: Author.

OCCUPATION-BASED
ACTIVITY ANALYSIS

SECTION

II

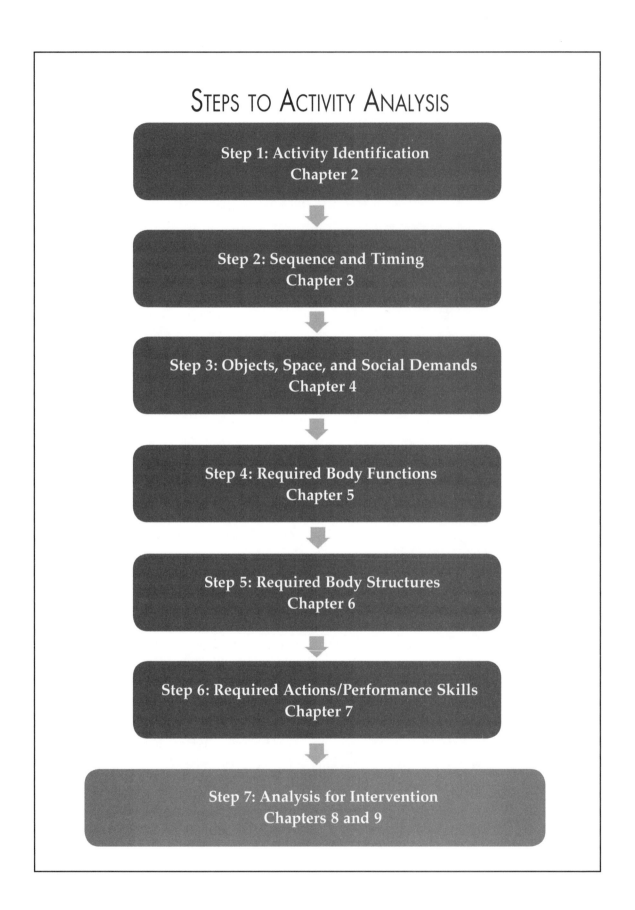

8

THE CLIENT

THE KEY TO CONDUCTING AN
OCCUPATION-BASED ACTIVITY ANALYSIS

OBJECTIVES

1. Understand what aspects of the client are key to conducting an occupation-based activity analysis.

2. Identify how client values, beliefs, and spirituality influence participation in occupations and activities.

3. List the information gathered during an occupational profile.

4. Explain how the client's physical, social, cultural, personal, temporal, and virtual contexts can influence performance in occupations and activities.

5. Understand how performance patterns such as habits, routines, rituals, and roles all influence participation in occupations and activities.

Activities can be examined from the perspective of the typical demands of activity or with the client's perspective or contexts in mind. Activities themselves do not lie in isolation but are woven into individual lives with distinct features and demands based on the physical and social environment the person performs the activity in. In order to understand the demands of an activity as a client needs and wants to do it, an occupation-based activity analysis must be completed. This chapter focuses on the unique characteristics of occupation-based activity analysis and how it is conducted. The activity demands are examined from the perspective of the objects and properties, space, social demands, sequence and timing, and actions the client uses to participate in

the occupation. It also examines the contexts that support or inhibit participation in the occupation. This includes examining the cultural, personal, temporal, virtual, physical, and social contexts. The client's interests, values, beliefs, and spirituality also influence elements of participation. The performance patterns, such as the habits, routines, rituals, and roles, may also play an important part in engaging in the occupation.

ACTIVITY DEMANDS REDEFINED

In order to understand how an occupation is defined by a client, each of the activity demands of the occupation the client needs or wants to do must be examined and how they manifest within the client's life. In order to do this, the process in which the activity analysis is conducted is slightly different, in that instead of understanding just an activity, you are becoming aware of the client and how he or she defines an occupation. In Chapter 1, the seven basic steps to an activity analysis were introduced. In an occupation-based activity analysis, step 1 becomes occupation awareness and requires a deeper analysis.

OCCUPATION AWARENESS

The first step to understanding an activity that has meaning to your client (an occupation) is to gain an understanding of how your client defines that occupation. In Chapter 2, the areas of occupation were defined as they are listed in the *Occupational Therapy*

Thomas, H. *Occupation-Based Activity Analysis* (pp. 141-157). © 2012 SLACK Incorporated

Practice Framework, 2nd Edition (Framework). There were multiple activities and tasks listed under the areas of activities of daily living (ADL), instrumental activities of daily living (IADL), rest and sleep, education, work, play, leisure, and social participation. As you may recall, some activities may be classified into several different areas of occupation, based on how the client defines them. For example, painting can be seen as a leisure activity or as work, based on why the client is painting. The first best step to an occupation-based activity analysis is asking the client to define the occupation he or she wants or needs to do. What defines successful participation for him or her? How does this occupation play a part in his or her life?

Understanding the occupation also requires understanding the person participating in the occupation—gaining knowledge of their values, beliefs, and spirituality. Values are defined as "principles, standards, or qualities considered worthwhile by the client" (American Occupational Therapy Association [AOTA], 2008, p. 633). Beliefs are ideas or concepts that the client deem to be true (AOTA, 2008). Beliefs and values influence how and why a person performs an occupation. A person who does not believe in using electricity to cook may perform cooking tasks differently. Values influence the standards to which a person will hold true when a decision must be made during an activity or the strength to which they put efforts toward certain steps. A person who values family may put forth a great amount of effort toward including all members of the family in an ancestry scrapbook. The spirituality of the person and the spiritual meaning the occupation has for the client can influence performance as well. Spirituality is related to how the client understands and seeks to gain "answers to ultimate questions about life, about meaning, and the sacred" (AOTA, 2008, p. 634). The guiding motivations to act during an occupation may come from spiritual motivation, derived meaning beyond money or tangible benefits. For example, a client may choose to volunteer for a homeless shelter because of the spiritual meaning it has for him or her, giving him or her a sense of purpose and fulfillment.

THE OCCUPATIONAL PROFILE

In order to gain an understanding of the client and the occupations that are important to him or her, the occupational therapy (OT) practitioner gathers this information through an occupational profile. The occupational profile is part of the evaluation process but does not necessarily only occur at the initiation of services. The profile is conducted through an interview of the client, client's family, caregivers, and

other significant people in his or her life. The purpose of the profile is to gain an understanding of the client's interests, values, needs, occupational history, patterns of daily living, and his or her priorities for outcomes (AOTA, 2008). Through the process of interviewing the client (and significant others), the OT practitioner should be able to determine the following:

+ Who the client is, including family, caregivers, etc.

+ Why the client is receiving OT services—what are his or her concerns with daily life activities.

+ Which areas of occupation he or she is having trouble with (as discussed in the previous paragraph), and which have been successful.

+ Which contexts support or inhibit participation in the occupation(s).

+ In what occupations the client has participated in the past, what he or she currently engages in, and what desired future occupations are.

+ What the client's priorities and chosen outcomes are (AOTA, 2008).

There is no set list of questions to ask the client in order to ask these questions, as the profile is a dynamically changing and interactive interview. The practitioner should actively listen to the client and base questions not only on the needed information but on the client's responses. Questioning the client about the occupations that are difficult will give you a basis on which to break down and analyze the occupation. Within the occupational profile process, information must also be gleamed about the client's contexts.

CONTEXTS

The Physical Context

Occupations take place within an environment that surrounds the client as well as in conditions that lie within the client. These contexts can either support or inhibit participation in an occupation. The external environment is called the *physical context* and includes all non-human objects and space. This includes both man-made and natural environments. It is important to understand the physical environment in which an occupation occurs, as this can influence demand for performance skills and body functions needed. The terrain, temperature, size, noise level, and lighting are all part of the physical context that should be considered as part of the space demands for the occupation (Figure 8-1). The objects that are part of the environment should also be considered, as their

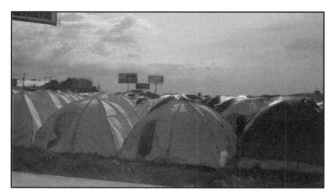

Figure 8-1. Example of how the environment can influence performance: the rubble-filled streets of Haiti impede residents' ability to navigate their community and conduct business.

placement, arrangement, and properties can also have an influence on participation. Buildings, plants, tables, tools, equipment, and furniture are examples of objects that are part of the physical context (AOTA, 2008). This information can be utilized to determine the objects and properties required for an occupation, as well as providing additional information about the objects surrounding the environment in which the occupation takes place.

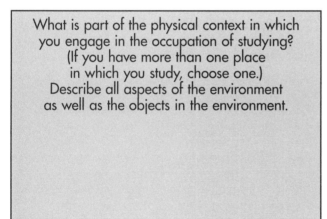

What is part of the physical context in which you engage in the occupation of studying? (If you have more than one place in which you study, choose one.) Describe all aspects of the environment as well as the objects in the environment.

The Social Context

The *social context* is made up of the people in the client's environments and the expectations of those people or groups (AOTA, 2008). The social context can include the client's friends, spouse, boyfriend/girlfriend, caregivers, coworkers, colleagues, or associations with organizations or groups of people. The relationship that the client has with individuals, groups, or organizations can provide a support or hindrance to participation in occupations. For example, a spouse can support a client's actions toward writing in a journal every day by giving him or her privacy and quiet during the client's writing time.

For a client who is trying to stop drinking alcohol, a group of friends can be a hindrance by offering alcoholic drinks to the client. Gaining awareness of the social contexts in which the client functions opens a window of understanding to the social demands of the occupations the client needs or wants to engage in.

The Cultural Context

The client's customs, behavior standards, and beliefs are shaped by their *cultural context*. Culture includes ethnicity, political environment, philosophy, and ethos of a work environment or organization that one is part of. Family traditions are part of the client's culture and determine roles as well as expectations of the client's actions. The laws and regulations that afford opportunities or limitations as well as personal rights are also considered part of the cultural context. This includes support and access to education, employment, and economic support (AOTA, 2008). How a person dresses, greets others, and acts toward strangers is set by cultural expectations and can change based on the cultural context one is in. For example, in France people greet each other by kissing each cheek, while in the United States people traditionally shake hands. Within organizations, a specific culture emerges with expectations and actions that are unique. For example, in one hospital there may be an expectation that all occupational therapists address sexuality with their clients, while in another hospital it is the psychologist who does this. Geographic areas may have a culture that determines attitudes and behaviors with the residents. For example, there are distinct cultural differences between residents of California and those of New York.

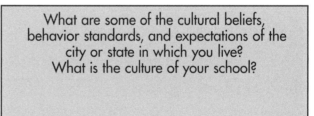

What are some of the cultural beliefs, behavior standards, and expectations of the city or state in which you live? What is the culture of your school?

The Personal Context

The *personal context* involves aspects of the person that are not health related but are still personal identifiers, such as age, gender, educational level, and socioeconomic status (AOTA, 2008). It is important to understand that disability or diagnosis is not part of the personal context. The personal context can apply to a personal role within an organization and what specific population a person belongs to. For example, the personal context of a client might be that he is a 62-year-old male who is a part-time employee of a construction company and is a Vietnam veteran. Understanding your client's personal context gives you a better understanding of the demands of the occupations they need to engage in. Age of the client may influence the type of occupation, how it is performed, and its complexity. For example, gardening for a 4-year-old may be very different from gardening for a 70-year-old. Socioeconomic level has an impact on multiple aspects of engagement in occupations, primarily access to needed space and objects. For example, a homeless man may have difficulty finding access to a computer to search job openings than a man who is middle income and has a computer in his home. The educational level of the client will reflect in his or her reading ability and access to certain opportunities. A woman without a high school diploma will have limited access to some occupations that require a high school diploma or higher educational level. As with all of the contexts, the personal context can support or inhibit participation in an occupation but can also provide needed information into the demands of the occupation.

Describe your personal context. This includes your age, gender, socioeconomic group, educational level, and what organizational or social status you may have.

The Temporal Context

Occupations occur within a space in time, which is the *temporal context*. Time is defined by stages of life, duration of actual time, time of day, rhythm of activity, or time of year. The temporal context can influence how an occupation is performed, when, and at what pace. For example, if the length of time available for a client to prepare a meal is very short, the demands are very different on the client than if he or she had hours to prepare. The stage of life a client is in may also change the demands of the occupation, as paying bills is very different for those in the early adulthood ages than for those at the end of life. The pattern and rhythm of occupations contributes to

the temporal aspects of an occupation. This includes the timing of steps, the repetition of certain aspects of the occupation, or how the occupation is weaved into a sequence of other occupations. Understanding the temporal context that surrounds and influences the occupation being analyzed allows the clinician to recognize how aspects of timing and placement of the occupation within the spectrum of time can influence the demands on the client. For example, if John typically wakes up at 9 a.m. to leave for work at 9:45, the clinician has an idea of what time of day John conducts his self care, as well as the amount of time he has to complete all of the self care tasks.

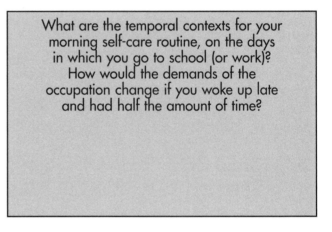

What are the temporal contexts for your morning self-care routine, on the days in which you go to school (or work)? How would the demands of the occupation change if you woke up late and had half the amount of time?

The Virtual Context

Communication occurring in the absence of physical contact occurs in the *virtual context*. This takes place through the use of computers, the Internet, cellular phones, telephones, video conferencing, and radio transmission (AOTA, 2008). The virtual context is an environment in which information can be sent and received without physical interaction with another. Advancements in technology have expanded access to this context to nearly anywhere, with portable devices such as cellular phones (Figure 8-2). A client can be supported or inhibited in their occupations by access or lack of access to the virtual context. A person who was recently diagnosed with multiple sclerosis can connect with others with the diagnosis through an online support group. A father coaching his son's baseball team may be interrupted by e-mail and text messages coming in on his cellular phone. The virtual context may or may not influence a client's desired occupation. Given the current use of technology and its immersion into daily life, the virtual context can be an embedded part of any occupation in which the client intermittently uses during another occupation. For example, a client may check her e-mail on her phone periodically while cooking dinner.

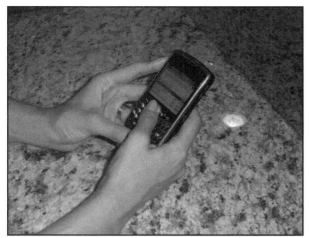

Figure 8-2. The virtual context also includes cellular phones.

> What virtual contexts are part of your daily occupations? What virtual contexts do you embed within other occupations?

PERFORMANCE PATTERNS

Performance patterns are the habits, routines, rituals, and roles that influence and surround participation in occupations. When analyzing an occupation, an essential step is to investigate the patterns in which the client engages and how they influence the demands of the occupation. Habits and routines can influence how and when an occupation is performed. This can be found to either be a support or hindrance to performance.

Habits

A *habit* is an automatic behavior or action that is part of functional patterns of everyday life (AOTA, 2008). Habits allow us to move and function on a more automatic basis. These habits emerge from repetition until the behaviors become automatic. While many habits allow us to function at a higher level and are useful, there are many habits that limit functioning and are termed *dominating*. A helpful habit would be to automatically shut and lock the door when leaving the house. A dominating habit would be chewing on fingernails while talking to a stranger or repeatedly washing hands after using the restroom. Understanding a client's habits will help the clinician evaluate the steps used to complete an occupation, as well as the timing and sequence of these steps. A client's habits may interfere with meeting the demands of the activity or may be a part of successful participation.

> What habits do you engage in which support your daily occupations? Are there any habits which you feel are dominating or inhibiting performance in daily occupations?

Routines

Routines are also part of performance patterns which provide structure for the flow of daily activities. Routines are patterns of behavior and actions that are regular and repetitive. These are sequences of tasks that are followed in order to complete an occupation. For example, before going to bed, many people have a series of activities they perform in order to prepare themselves for sleep. At the end of the day when the body and mind are often tired, it is helpful to follow a usual routine. Routines are often influenced by cultural and ecological contexts (AOTA, 2008). While interviewing the client during the occupational profile process, it is helpful to ask the client about his or her daily routines. This gives the clinician a chance to understand how certain occupations lead into others and the place each takes in the structure of the client's life.

Rituals

Humans perform actions that have cultural, spiritual, or social meaning called *rituals*. These rituals are part of a person's identity, value system, and beliefs. Rituals often stem from cultural or social traditions or symbolic actions as part of a belief system such as a religion. For example, a family may have a ritual of having the smallest child place the star on the top of the Christmas tree (Figure 8-3). A couple may have a nightly ritual of praying together before going to sleep. Rituals have meaning and contribute to those who are part of the social or cultural group who engages in the events and actions that comprise the rituals. The way in which these rituals are performed will be unique to each client; thus, it is important to understand their place in daily occupations.

Roles

The behaviors and actions expected of a client by the social and cultural contexts in which they are immersed define the *roles* that the client encompasses. A client can define and clarify what those roles are, as well as the occupations that each role entails. A client can identify with several roles within his or her life in many different contexts. For example, within the family, Jenifer is mother, daughter, sister, and wife. At work she is a public relations director, a confidant to her employer, and a coworker. As a member of her community, she is a member of her city council. In her social context, she is a friend. Understanding the client's roles helps identify the occupations he or she is expected to desire to engage in. It also gives perspective to the social demands on the client for the occupations which correspond to certain roles. For example, if your client is a mother of triplets, this gives a deeper understanding to the occupations she must engage in as her role of mother.

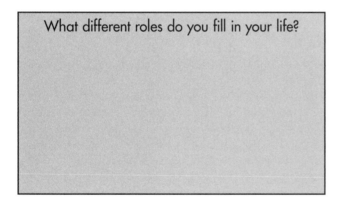

What different roles do you fill in your life?

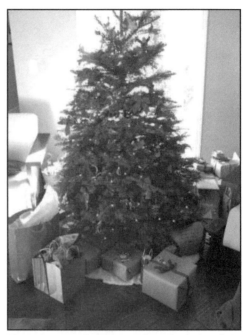

Figure 8-3. An example of a ritual is decorating a Christmas tree.

Conclusion

Conducting an occupation-based activity analysis involves gaining an understanding of how the client defines the occupation and the multiple contexts that surround them. The process of occupation-based analysis runs parallel to that of an activity analysis but adds in components of evaluating the client's meaning and purpose for engaging in the occupation as well as the performance patterns and the contexts that support or hinder participation. All of this information can be gathered through the occupational profile interview at the initiation of services or as the therapy relationship expands. Through an occupation-based activity analysis, the clinician has a better understanding of how occupations can be used therapeutically and how open the client is to adaptations. This process will be discussed in the next chapter.

Activities

1. Assess how each of your contexts either supports or inhibits your performance in studying. Using Activity 8-1, give a brief description in each corresponding box as appropriate. If a context neither inhibits nor supports performance, leave that box empty.

2. Over the next week, use the grid given to record each activity that you do throughout the day. Write down what you do each hour of every day. Do not go into too much detail, but list a one- or two-word description for each hour (grid is shown in Activity 8-2).

   At the end of the week, refer back to your list of roles. Using colored pencils or pens, indicate one color for each role. Go through the week of activities, and highlight each activity according to what role that activity corresponds. You do not have to highlight each activity.

   Is most of your time dedicated to one role?

   Is there a role you wish had more of on your schedule?

   How would this look different if you were to suddenly become ill?

3. Using the activity analysis form provided (Activity 8-3), complete an analysis of an occupation that is meaningful to you.

Activity 8-1

Context	Supports	Inhibits
Physical		
Social		
Cultural		
Personal		
Temporal		
Virtual		

QUESTIONS

1. Why is it important to find out a client's values and beliefs?

2. Using the example of washing hair in the shower, in what ways could an occupation-based activity analysis be different than an activity analysis?

3. What are examples of activities that can be spiritual but not religious?

4. In what ways can an occupational profile be obtained for a client who is unable to speak?

5. Your client Donny is an 82-year-old man who lives in a nursing home. He has a pet parrot and his primary goal is to be able to feed and give water to the parrot in his cage twice a day as the nursing staff are not allowed to touch the cage. What are the physical, social, temporal, and cultural contexts to be considered?

6. How are roles, routines, habits, and rituals different from each other? How might they be inter-related?

REFERENCES

American Occupational Therapy Association. (2008). Occupational therapy practice framework: Domain and process, 2nd edition. *American Journal of Occupational Therapy, 62*(6), 609-639.

Activity 8-2

Time	Monday	Tuesday	Wednesday	Thursday	Friday	Saturday	Sunday
6:00 a.m.							
7:00 a.m.							
8:00 a.m.							
9:00 a.m.							
10:00 a.m.							
11:00 a.m.							
Noon							
1:00 p.m.							
2:00 p.m.							
3:00 p.m.							
4:00 p.m.							
5:00 p.m.							
6:00 p.m.							
7:00 p.m.							
8:00 p.m.							
9:00 p.m.							
10:00 p.m.							
11:00 p.m.							
Midnight							
Later							

Activity 8-3

OCCUPATION-BASED ACTIVITY ANALYSIS FORM

Complete the following occupation-based activity analysis on an occupation that is meaningful to you.

1. Occupation: _____

Area(s) of occupation for the client:	Subcategory:
Activities of daily living	_____
Instrumental activities of daily living	_____
Education	_____
Work	_____
Play	_____
Leisure	_____
Social participation	_____

2. Values, beliefs, spirituality associated with participation:

3. Contexts: Indicate how each supports or inhibits your participation in this occupation.

Context	Supports	Inhibits
Physical/space demands		
Social		
Cultural		
Personal		
Temporal		
Virtual		

4. Objects and their properties required:

5. Social demands:

6. Sequence and timing:

1. _____
2. _____
3. _____
4. _____
5. _____
6. _____
7. _____
8. _____
9. _____
10. _____

(continued)

Activity 8-3 (continued)

OCCUPATION-BASED ACTIVITY ANALYSIS FORM

7. Body Functions Required:

Function	Required? Check If Yes	How It Is Used
Judgment		
Concept formation		
Metacognition		
Cognitive flexibility		
Insight/awareness		
Sustained attention		
Selective attention		
Divided attention		
Short-term memory		
Working memory		
Long-term memory		
Discrimination of senses: Auditory		
Discrimination of senses: Tactile		
Discrimination of senses: Visual		
Discrimination of senses: Olfactory		
Discrimination of senses: Vestibular-proprioception		
Multisensory processing		
Sensory memory		
Spatial relationships		
Temporal relationships		
Recognition		
Categorization		
Generalization		
Awareness of reality		
Logical/coherent thought		
Appropriate thought content		
Execution of learned movements		
Coping		
Behavioral regulation		
Body image		
Self-concept		
Self-esteem		
Arousal		
Consciousness		
Orientation to self		
Orientation to place		
Orientation to time		
Orientation to others		
Emotional stability		
Motivation		

(continued)

Activity 8-3 (continued)

OCCUPATION-BASED ACTIVITY ANALYSIS FORM

Function	Required? Check If Yes	How It Is Used
Impulse control		
Appetite		
Sleep		
Detection/registration		
Visual modulation		
Integration of senses		
Awareness at distances		
Tolerance of ambient sounds		
Location and distance of sounds		
Moving against gravity		
Taste		
Smell		
Body in space		
Comfort with touch		
Localizing pain		
Thermal awareness		
Joint range of motion		
Joint stability/alignment		
Strength		
Muscle tone		
Muscle endurance		
Stretch reflex		
ATNR		
STNR		
Righting and supporting reflex		
Eye–hand coordination		
Eye–foot coordination		
Bilateral coordination		
Crossing midline		
Fine motor control		
Gross motor control		
Oculomotor control		
Gait patterns		
Blood pressure		
Heart rate		
Respiratory rate		
Respiratory rhythm		
Respiratory depth		
Physical endurance, aerobic capacity		
Voice functions		
Voice rhythm and fluency		

(continued)

Activity 8-3 (continued)

OCCUPATION-BASED ACTIVITY ANALYSIS FORM

Function	Required? Check If Yes	How It Is Used
Alternative vocalization		
Digestive system		
Metabolic system		
Endocrine system		
Urinary functions		
Genital and reproductive functions		
Protective functions of the skin		
Repair functions of the skin		

8. Muscular analysis of movements required:

Muscle	Required? Check If Yes
Shoulder flexion	
Shoulder extension	
Shoulder abduction	
Shoulder adduction	
Shoulder internal rotation	
Shoulder external rotation	
Elbow flexion	
Elbow extension	
Wrist supination	
Wrist pronation	
Wrist flexion	
Wrist extension	
Thumb flexion	
Thumb abduction	
Finger flexion	
Finger extension	
Trunk flexion	
Trunk extension	
Trunk rotation	
Lower extremities	

9. Body structures required:

Category	Body Structure	Required? Check If Yes
Nervous system	Frontal lobe	
	Temporal lobe	
	Parietal lobe	
	Occipital lobe	
	Midbrain	

(continued)

Activity 8-3 (continued)

OCCUPATION-BASED ACTIVITY ANALYSIS FORM

Category	Body Structure	Required? Check If Yes
Nervous system (continued)	Diencephalon	
	Basal ganglia	
	Cerebellum	
	Brain stem	
	Cranial nerves	
	Spinal cord	
	Spinal nerves	
	Meninges	
	Sympathetic nervous system	
	Parasympathetic nervous system	
Eyes, ears, and related structures	Eyeball: Conjunctiva, cornea, iris, retina, lens, vitreous body	
	Structures around eye: Lachrimal gland, eyelid, eyebrow, external ocular muscles	
	Structure of external ear	
	Structure of middle ear: Tympanic membrane, eustachian canal, ossicles	
	Structures of inner ear: Cochlea, vestibular labyrinth, semicircular canals, internal auditory meatus	
Voice and speech structures	Structures of the nose: External nose, nasal septum, nasal fossae	
	Structure of the mouth: Teeth, gums, hard palate, soft palate, tongue, lips	
	Structure of pharynx: Nasal pharynx and oral pharynx	
	Structure of larynx: Vocal folds	
Cardiovascular system	Heart: Atria, ventricles	
	Arteries	
	Veins	
	Capillaries	
Immune system	Lymphatic vessels	
	Lymphatic nodes	
	Thymus	
	Spleen	
	Bone marrow	
Respiratory system	Trachea	
	Lungs: Bronchial tree, alveoli	
	Thoracic cage	
	Muscles of respiration: Intercostal muscles, diaphragm	
Digestive, metabolic, and endocrine systems	Salivary glands	
	Esophagus	

(continued)

Activity 8-3 (continued)

OCCUPATION-BASED ACTIVITY ANALYSIS FORM

Category	*Body Structure*	*Required?* *Check If Yes*
Digestive, metabolic, and endocrine systems (continued)	Stomach	
	Intestines: Small and large	
	Pancreas	
	Liver	
	Gall bladder and ducts	
	Endocrine glands: Pituitary, thyroid, parathyroid, adrenal	
Genitourinary and reproductive systems	Urinary system: Kidneys, ureters, bladder, urethra	
	Structure of pelvic floor	
	Structure of reproductive system: Ovaries, uterus, breast and nipple, vagina and external genitalia, testes, penis, prostate	
Structures related to movement	Bones of cranium	
	Bones of face	
	Bones of neck region	
	Joints of head and neck	
	Bones of shoulder region	
	Joints of shoulder region	
	Muscles of shoulder region	
	Bones of upper arm	
	Elbow joint	
	Muscles of upper arm	
	Ligaments and fascia of upper arm	
	Bones of forearm	
	Wrist joint	
	Muscles of forearm	
	Ligaments and fascia of forearm	
	Bones of hand	
	Joints of hand and fingers	
	Muscles of hand	
	Ligaments and fascia of hand	
	Bones of pelvic region	
	Joints of pelvic region	
	Muscles of pelvic region	
	Ligaments and fascia of pelvic region	
	Bones of thigh	
	Hip joint	
	Muscles of thigh	
	Ligaments and fascia of thigh	

(continued)

Activity 8-3 (continued)

OCCUPATION-BASED ACTIVITY ANALYSIS FORM

Category	Body Structure	Required? Check If Yes
Structures related to movement (continued)	Bones of lower leg	
	Knee joint	
	Muscles of lower leg	
	Ligaments and fascia of lower leg	
	Bones of ankle and foot	
	Ankle, foot, and toe joints	
	Muscle of ankle and foot	
	Ligaments of fascia of ankle and foot	
	Cervical vertebral column	
	Lumbar vertebral column	
	Sacral vertebral column	
	Coccyx	
	Muscles of trunk	
	Ligaments and fascia of trunk	
Skin and related structures	Areas of skin: Head, neck, shoulder, upper extremity, pelvic region, lower extremities, trunk, and back	
	Structure of skin glands: Sweat and sebaceous	
	Structure of nails: Fingernails and toenails	
	Structure of hair	

10. Performance skills required:

Skill	Required? Check If Yes	How the Skill Is Used
Motor/praxis		
Sensory (perceptual)		
Emotional regulation		
Cognitive		
Communication/social		

(continued)

Activity 8-3 (continued)

OCCUPATION-BASED ACTIVITY ANALYSIS FORM

11. Performance patterns:

Parts of this occupation has elements of which of the following: (check all that apply)

✓	Pattern	Describe
	Useful habit	
	Dominating habit	
	Routine	
	Ritual	
	Role	

ex: murder ball movie

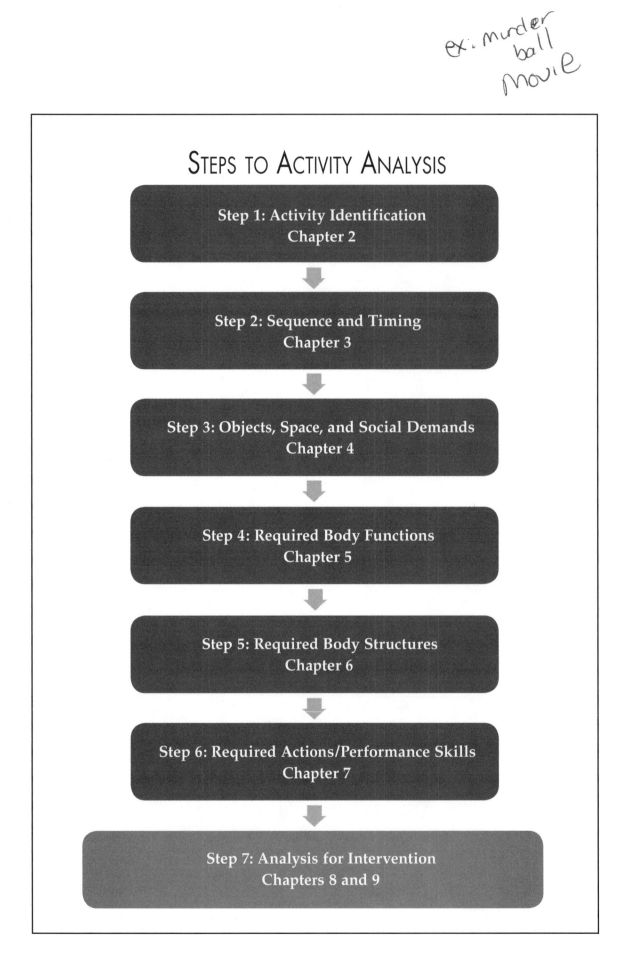

STEPS TO ACTIVITY ANALYSIS

Step 1: Activity Identification
Chapter 2

Step 2: Sequence and Timing
Chapter 3

Step 3: Objects, Space, and Social Demands
Chapter 4

Step 4: Required Body Functions
Chapter 5

Step 5: Required Body Structures
Chapter 6

Step 6: Required Actions/Performance Skills
Chapter 7

Step 7: Analysis for Intervention
Chapters 8 and 9

9

GRADING AND ADAPTING

OBJECTIVES

1. Define what grading of an activity means and how it is used in occupational therapy (OT).

2. Describe how to grade and activity up or down and when each is relevant.

3. Understand the concept of scaffolding and how it is used in OT practice.

4. Identify how to adapt activities and occupations in each of the activity demand areas.

5. Understand how adapting and grading of activities are used to reach common outcomes in OT practice.

One of the unique contributions that OT brings to health care is the use of occupations as an intervention modality and the ability to adapt those occupations to allow for greater participation in daily life activities. Changing an occupation can be done in several ways—by grading, scaffolding, or adapting. How and why an occupation is changed in some way depends on the overall goal of intervention and the theoretical approach the clinician is taking. This chapter will introduce the foundational reasons OT clinicians utilize grading, scaffolding, and adapting and how to use activity analysis principle to implement these approaches.

GRADING

The term *grading* often gets confused with the term *adapting*, and understandably so. Grading of an activity is used to increase or decrease the activity demands on the person while he or she is performing an activity. This is done incrementally, to provide the "just-right challenge" and allow the person to develop the skills he or she needs, while still assuring him or her success at completing the activity. Grading down an activity is done by making the activity easier or providing assistance at difficult points as to allow for success. Grading an activity down can be done by changing aspects of the activity demands, depending on where the client has difficulty. For example, if a child has difficulty with handwriting, we can grade down the activity by having him start with writing very large letters on paper with large lines. As he improves, we would grade up the activity by having him write smaller letters with smaller lines. To better understand the concepts of "grade up" and "grade down" think of the "steep grade" signs you see on the highway (Figure 9-1). If the grade is going down, the truck does not need to work as hard. Thus, if you grade down an activity, the client does not struggle as much. If the grade is going uphill, the truck will struggle and work hard to get to the top of the hill. If you grade up an activity, you are making it more difficult (if you are looking to provide more of a challenge to your client).

Grading up an activity is often done in OT practice in order provide a greater challenge to the client. For example, a client who is able to count out the correct

Thomas, H. *Occupation-Based Activity Analysis* (pp. 159-166).
© 2012 SLACK Incorporated

Figure 9-1. Grading can be compared to the grade of a hill.

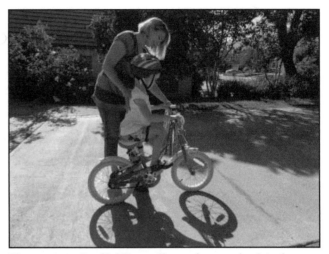

Figure 9-2. Scaffolding allows for gradual independence.

change for an item does well when completing the task in the quiet environment of a therapy session, so the clinician can grade up the activity by having him or her do the activity while in a noisy grocery store. This is an appropriate way to grade up an activity, as it matches the client's goals. Caution should be made when grading up an activity so that it does not cause undue struggle for the client, with little ties to desired outcomes. For example, if a client is working on being able to put books up on a bookshelf, to make the activity more difficult, a clinician could put weights around his or her wrists. True, this is making the task more difficult, but the clinician should question the use of this and whether it is causing undue struggle and taking away from the point of the activity. Care should also be taken with not grading up too many aspects of the activity at one time. Providing the "just-right challenge" requires understanding what will provide a challenge to the client, while still allowing them to be successful and not too frustrated. Think about how frustrated you would be if one of your teachers decided to grade up an assignment not by adding one addition piece to the assignment but by adding multiple parts. The same is true for your clients—they may become frustrated if too many additional challenges are added all at one time.

SCAFFOLDING

Scaffolding is a method of grading an activity by providing assistance to the client at times that he or she might struggle or be unable to successfully complete a step. Think of when a child is beginning to learn how to feed him- or herself. The parent will hold his or her hand over the little hand that is holding the spoon. At first, the parent must guide the child's hand

in scooping the food and bringing it to the mouth. Eventually, some of the support and assistance can be taken away when the child learns to bring the spoon to the mouth but continues to need help scooping the food. Little by little, the support (or scaffolding) is removed until the child is successful at completing the task on his or her own (albeit a bit messy). In this way, the activity begins as graded down but is slowly graded up as more challenge is given to the child and less to the parent. This technique is used frequently in OT sessions, as a client learns or relearns an occupation. An example of this is when a person who has had a stroke must relearn how to put on a shirt, perhaps with the use of only one arm. As the person begins to learn how to do this activity, the clinician may need to provide a great amount of assistance in order for the client to get the shirt on. As the client learns how to do the activity, the clinician will provide fewer cues and less assistance to allow the client to become more independent. The clinician will need to carefully think about the amount of assistance given and be sure that with each trial, the scaffolding (or amount of support) is slowly taken away (Figure 9-2).

HOW TO GRADE AN ACTIVITY

Grading an activity begins with a good understanding of the activity demands. What are the objects and properties being used? Can those be changed and made easier to use (or more difficult)? Can aspects of the environment be changed, such as the noise, temperature, working surface, or seating surface? How about the sequence and timing? Can the steps be changed or done in a different way? Perhaps

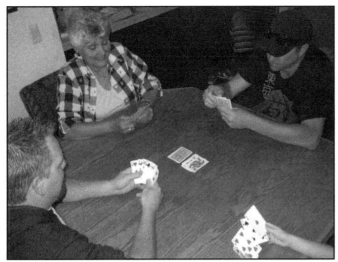

Figure 9-3. The activity of playing cards is one that may be graded up.

Activity 9-1

Describe how you would grade the activity of gardening by listing what you would change in each aspect of the activity demands.

Activity Demand	Grade Down	Grade Up
Objects and properties		
Space demands		
Social demands		
Sequence and timing		

---

the timing can be changed, allowing for more or less time to complete the activity. The social demands of an activity can be lessened by removing or changing rules of the activity or decreasing the expectations of others. For example, Brent is having a hard time playing board games with others. His occupational therapist grades the activity down so that he can re-learn how to participate in this occupation. She begins by having him play a simple game of solitaire, where there are no social demands on him by others. She grades up by having him play a card game with her. She further grades up by adding another player to the game. As Brent improves, she adds social demands such as rule of behavior and interactions with the players (Figure 9-3).

To grade an activity, think first of what areas of the activity demands the client is struggling with. Is there a great amount of joint mobility of the hands required but the client has limited range of motion? Having an understanding of how each of the activity demands will affect your client *before* he or she starts the activity will allow you to create ways to grade down the activity and allow him or her to be successful. Once you have identified the required actions that the client will have difficulty with, you

can choose to grade the activity down by providing scaffolding, changing the objects and properties, space demands, social demands, or sequence and timing. You can change the actions and skill level required by changing some of these activity demands or by providing assistance.

Use Activity 9-1 to practice grading an activity.

ADAPTING

Adapting an activity is changing or modifying an aspect of the activity to allow for successful participation in an occupation (Crepeau & Schell, 2009). Adaptation requires thinking differently about an activity and finding an alternative way of getting it done. This requires flexibility on the part of the clinician and the client. While similar to grading in that we are changing aspects of the activity demands, when adapting an activity, it is not with the intent to reduce or increase the demands on the client. The overall goal of adapting is to allow for greater participation and independence. This could also include teaching compensatory techniques and having him or her complete the activity differently

Activity 9-2

Adapt the activity of making scrambled eggs by modifying aspects of the following activity demands.

Activity Demand	Adaptation/Modification
Objects and properties	
Space demands	
Social demands	
Sequence and timing	

(changing the sequence and timing). Modifying the amount of support and cues in the environment, such as providing visual cues or reminders, is also a way to adapt to allow for greater success.

An example of adapting is if a clinician provides a spoon with a built-up handle that allows someone with severe arthritis be able to feed him or herself. If we go back to the example we used earlier of the child that is struggling with handwriting, we can adapt certain aspects of the activity to allow him to be more successful immediately. We can change the height of the desk and chair he sits in (space demands) or give him a pencil with a bigger grip (objects and properties). The choice to adapt an activity is fed by many different factors, including the client's desired outcomes, openness to change, and diagnosis; time limitations; and the clinician's theoretical perspective. A clinician who has only one session with a client may choose to teach the client how to adapt an activity to allow for greater independence immediately. The same is true of a client who has a progressive disease or one in which the current body functions and structures will not improve. The clinician may choose to adapt activities if the client's skill level is not likely to improve.

Use Activity 9-2 to practice modifying an activity.

OUTCOMES AND THE USE OF GRADING AND ADAPTING

Table 10 of the *Occupational Therapy Practice Framework, 2nd Edition* (*Framework*) (American Occupational Therapy Association [AOTA], 2008) defines nine broad outcomes of OT intervention: occupational performance, adaptation, health and wellness, participation, prevention, quality of life, role competence, self-advocacy, and occupational justice. The desired outcome for a client helps determine what approach the clinician should take.

Occupational Performance

Improving or enhancing *occupational performance* is one of the leading outcomes for OT practice. It is used when there is an inability to perform needed occupations or a limitation in being able to perform or if performance could be improved. This applies to a broad spectrum of diagnoses and populations. A person who has had a stroke and lost the use of the right arm may work toward regaining the ability to dress and bathe themselves. A woman with schizophrenia may work to improve social interaction skills. Grading and scaffolding of activities is very often utilized with this approach to gradually improve a person's ability to complete activities on their own. Changes in occupational performance stem from improvements in performance skills, body functions, habits, or routines.

Adaptation

When the client is unable to perform or is having difficulty performing an occupation, part or multiple parts of the activity demands can be modified, which leads to an outcome of adaptation. This outcome requires making changes and doing things differently. The focus of this outcome is on the clinician's and client's creative redesign of the activity demands. Modification or adaptation can be done on the objects and properties, space demands, social demands, sequence and timing, required actions, required body functions, or required body structures. Modifying one or more of these aspects would be part of the intervention process, with the eventual outcome being adaptation of the desired occupation.

Health and Wellness

Health and wellness are outcomes that have been separately defined but aptly put together as an outcome measure. *Health* is defined as "a state of physical, mental, and social well-being, as well as a positive concept emphasizing social and person resources and physical capacities" (AOTA, 2008,

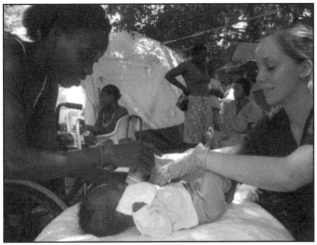

Figure 9-4. An occupational therapy student teaches infant-mother bonding techniques.

p. 662). As an outcome, it means that OT practitioners help clients reach a state of not only physical well-being and optimal use of physical abilities but to also reach a positive mental and social state. Achieving wellness occurs when mental/physical status is balanced and fit. This does not mean there is a lack of disease or disorder but that the client actively chooses to live a full and flourishing life. Health and wellness as an outcome is utilized with those who have a disability or illness as well as those who do not. An example of this type of outcome would be a recently retired man taking lessons to learn to play the piano, something he has always wanted to do. Modifying or adapting habits and routines can be part of the intervention process leading to this outcome. Activity analysis principles can be used in order to identify those activities that will lead to a greater sense of well-being for the client.

Participation

Simply put, *participation* as an outcome is the act of doing an occupation. Getting a client to engage in occupations that are meaningful and personally satisfying can be an outcome for intervention. Again, this outcome does not apply to only those with a disability or illness but to all people in which actually engaging in a meaningful occupation is a goal. An example of this would be to have a busy working father spend time playing baseball with his son.

Prevention

Prevention as an outcome focuses on promoting those things that may impede a healthy life. As the opponent of illness and injury, health as a preventative measure is created out of several factors at a personal, social, and environmental level. The *Framework* uses the following as the determinants

of health: "peace, shelter, education, food, income, a stable ecosystem, sustainable resources, social justice, and equity" (Kronenberg, Algado, & Pollard, 2005, p. 441). Preventing decline in any of these areas at a personal or societal level requires the OT practitioner to be able to analyze occupations and understand the complex interaction between the environment, human occupations, and performance. In order to promote a healthy lifestyle, the environment, objects, or actions required may need to be modified or adapted, changing aspects of how occupations are performed, the space or materials utilized, or the actions required. An example of this would be an educational support group for the caregivers of those with Alzheimer's disease to promote peace and physical well-being and prevent illness or familial unrest at home. This may include providing suggestions on how to adapt the home or tasks to decrease frustrations and safety hazards.

Quality of Life

Improved *quality of life* as an OT outcome involves understanding the client's perceived satisfaction with life, hope, self-concept, and overall health and functioning (AOTA, 2008). Life satisfaction is a person's perception of "progress toward one's goals" (AOTA, 2008, p. 663). Having hope is the belief that reaching a goal is possible. A person's self-concept is what he or she believes to be true about and overall feelings toward him- or herself. The first thing that people often associate with quality of life is health and functioning, which is not only physical health, but also the ability to complete self care and provide for oneself through work (AOTA, 2008). Achieving this as an outcome can be demonstrated in a multitude of ways, from providing a workshop environment for mentally retarded adolescents to begin work skills to summer day camps for children with working parents.

Role Competence

Roles are the set of behaviors that are expected by society or culture, based on the position the person has within familial or social contexts (AOTA, 2008). A person may play many different roles in her daily life, such as mother, student, wife, church member, and daughter. Meeting *role competence* is the ability to "effectively meet the demands of roles in which the client engages" (AOTA, 2008, p. 663). An example of this would be if a mother with depression implements bonding techniques with her baby (see Figure 9-4). Role competence can be enabled by adapting activities to allow for greater ability to fulfill roles. For example, a worker may adapt his work station so that there are fewer distractions, as to improve his productivity at work (his role as an employee).

Activity 9-3

Aspect	Adaptation	Adaptation
Sequence and timing		
Objects and properties		
Space demands		
Social demands		
Body functions		
Performance skills		

Self-Advocacy

Self-advocacy occurs when a person advocates and promotes his or her own strengths, needs, goals, or legal rights and responsibilities. Advocating for oneself includes not only having an understanding of these things but being able to communicate these aspects to others. This requires the person to have an understanding of him- or herself and how it relates to the contexts in which he or she engages. For example, a woman with a disability speaks to her employer when she is overlooked several times when opportunities for advancement have come up. Another example of where activity analysis principles are used is when a young man with a recent spinal cord injury manages and dictates how his caregivers complete his self care. The client must learn how to break down tasks into concise steps in order to direct his care.

Occupational Justice

Occupational justice refers to the right that all people must have access to and be able to participate in occupations that are meaningful to them. All humans should have access to those occupations that satisfy health, societal, and personal needs. For many, this means having access to resources or being allowed inclusion into social contexts. For example, men and women in prisons have very little access to occupations that provide any personal meaning to them. An example of an occupational justice outcome would be the establishment of a free computer lab with adapted computer keyboards and mouse alternatives for those with disabilities to be able to use the Internet.

CONCLUSION

Changing aspects of an activity to meet the client's needs is a fundamental function of OT practitioners. Changes can be made to make the activity easier and allow the client immediate performance or can be graded up slowly to allow for an increase in skill level. While grading of activities is primarily utilized when the desired outcome is occupational performance, it can be seen in all of the other types of outcomes as well. Through each of the types, adaptation can be found. Being able to see an activity from all aspects allows the clinician to find different ways it can be done. Modifying one aspect of an activity can address multiple outcomes. If a woman who uses a wheelchair has a baby who ends up in the neonatal intensive care unit, the occupational therapist can coach her to self-advocate for an adapted baby incubator, so that she is able to reach inside and hold her baby. With the adaptation of the incubator, she has met adaptation, health and wellness, participation, quality of life, role competence, self-advocacy, and occupational justice outcomes.

ACTIVITY

1. How would you adapt the activity of washing hair in the shower for limitations in the following body functions:

   Decreased joint mobility in the shoulder

   Decreased bilateral coordination

   Low vision

   Decreased fine motor

   Decreased memory

2. Using Activity 9-3, list two ways each of the activity demands of washing hair in the shower can be adapted.

3. Choose six different activities and set up a station for each, with all of the materials needed for each activity. Example of activities are playing a board game, washing windows, brushing teeth, making tea, and writing a letter to be sent in the mail. At each station, place a piece

of paper. On the left side of the paper, write "adaptation" and on the right, write "aspect." The students are to break up into groups and each to go to a station. They will be given one minute to brainstorm a way to adapt the activity. They will write it down on the sheet and then indicate what they are adapting: objects and properties used, the space, required actions, or social demands. They are to only write down one idea for adapting the activity. Once one minute has passed, the groups are to shift over to a different station and come up with a new idea for how to adapt the activity. Each group must read what has already been written down in order to not duplicate ideas. Once a group is unable to create a new idea, they are out of the game.

4. Make a list of ways in which to adapt the activity of washing hair in the shower. What aspects of the activity demands are you adapting?

QUESTIONS

1. What is the difference between grading and adapting?

2. At what times would it be appropriate to adapt an activity?

3. List the top 10 challenged body functions utilized when riding a bike. How would you adapt for each of these?

4. What are ways you might see scaffolding occurring with adults (not in a therapy setting)?

REFERENCES

American Occupational Therapy Association. (2008). Occupational therapy practice framework: Domain and process (2nd ed.). *American Journal of Occupational Therapy, 62,* 625–683.

Crepeau, E., & Schell, B. (2009). Analyzing occupations and activity. In E. Crepeau, E. Cohn, & B. Boyt Schell (Eds.), *Willard and Spackman's occupational therapy* (11th ed., pp. 359–374). Philadelphia, PA: Lippincott Williams & Wilkins.

Kroeneberg, F., Algado, S. S., & Pollard, N. (2005). *Occupational therapy without borders: Learning from the spirit of survivors.* Philadelphia, PA: Elsevier/Churchill Livingstone.

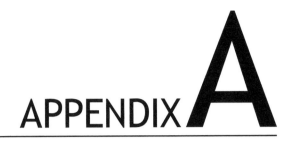

BLANK FORMS AND ACTIVITIES

BLANK FORMS AND ACTIVITIES INCLUDED IN THIS APPENDIX

Occupation-Based Activity Analysis Form

Muscular Analysis

Required Body Functions Analysis

Performance Skills Analysis

Thomas, H. *Occupation-Based Activity Analysis* (pp. 167-172).
© 2012 SLACK Incorporated

Occupation-Based Activity Analysis Form

Complete the following occupation-based activity analysis on an occupation that is meaningful to you.

1. Occupation: _____

Area(s) of occupation for the client:	Subcategory:
Activities of daily living	_____
Instrumental activities of daily living	_____
Education	_____
Work	_____
Play	_____
Leisure	_____
Social participation	_____

2. Values, beliefs, spirituality associated with participation:

3. Contexts: Indicate how each supports or inhibits your participation in this occupation.

Context	Supports	Inhibits
Physical/space demands		
Social		
Cultural		
Personal		
Temporal		
Virtual		

4. Objects and their properties required:

5. Social demands:

6. Sequence and timing:

   1. _____
   2. _____
   3. _____
   4. _____
   5. _____
   6. _____
   7. _____
   8. _____
   9. _____
   10. _____

MUSCULAR ANALYSIS

Complete a muscular analysis of getting a snack out of a vending machine.

Muscle	Not Used	Minimally Challenged	Greatly Challenged
Shoulder flexion			
Shoulder extension			
Shoulder abduction			
Shoulder adduction			
Shoulder internal rotation			
Shoulder external rotation			
Elbow flexion			
Elbow extension			
Wrist supination			
Wrist pronation			
Wrist flexion			
Wrist extension			
Thumb flexion			
Thumb abduction			
Finger flexion			
Finger extension			
Trunk flexion			
Trunk extension			
Trunk rotation			
Lower extremities			

REQUIRED BODY FUNCTIONS ANALYSIS

Function	How It Is Used	None	Minimally Challenged	Greatly Challenged
Judgment				
Concept formation				
Metacognition				
Cognitive flexibility				
Insight/awareness				
Sustained attention				
Selective attention				
Divided attention				
Short-term memory				
Long-term memory				
Working memory				
Discrimination of senses: Auditory				
Discrimination of senses: Tactile				
Discrimination of senses: Visual				
Discrimination of senses: Olfactory				
Discrimination of senses: Vestibular-proprioception				
Multisensory processing				
Sensory memory				
Spatial relationships				
Temporal relationships				
Recognition				
Categorization				
Generalization				
Awareness of reality				
Logical/coherent thought				
Appropriate thought content				
Execution of learned movements				
Coping				
Behavioral regulation				
Body image				
Self-concept				
Self-esteem				
Arousal				
Consciousness				
Orientation to self				
Orientation to place				
Orientation to time				
Orientation to others				
Emotional stability				
Motivation				
Impulse control				
Appetite				
Sleep				

(continued)

Function	How It Is Used	None	Minimally Challenged	Greatly Challenged
Detection/registration				
Visual modulation				
Integration of senses				
Awareness at distances				
Tolerance of ambient sounds				
Location and distance of sounds				
Moving against gravity				
Taste				
Smell				
Body in space				
Comfort with touch				
Localizing pain				
Thermal awareness				
Joint range of motion				
Joint stability/alignment				
Strength				
Muscle tone				
Muscle endurance				
Stretch reflex				
ATNR				
STNR				
Righting and supporting reflex				
Eye–hand coordination				
Eye–foot coordination				
Bilateral coordination				
Crossing midline				
Fine motor control				
Gross motor control				
Oculomotor control				
Gait patterns				
Blood pressure				
Heart rate				
Respiratory rate				
Respiratory rhythm				
Respiratory depth				
Physical endurance, aerobic capacity				
Voice functions				
Voice rhythm and fluency				
Alternative vocalization				
Digestive system				
Metabolic system				
Endocrine system				
Urinary functions				
Genital and reproductive functions				
Protective functions of the skin				
Repair functions of the skin				

PERFORMANCE SKILLS ANALYSIS

Skill	None	Low	Mod	High	Examples of how the skill is used
Motor/praxis					
Sensory (perceptual)					
Emotional regulation					
Cognitive					
Communication/social					

BLANK ACTIVITY ANALYSIS FORMS

BLANK ACTIVITY ANALYSIS FORMS IN THIS APPENDIX

Activity Analysis Form

Occupation-Based Activity Analysis Form

Thomas, H. *Occupation-Based
Activity Analysis* (pp. 173-182)
© 2011 SLACK Incorporated

Activity Analysis Form

1. Occupation:

Area(s) of occupation for the client: Subcategory:

- ☐ Activities of daily living
- ☐ Instrumental activities of daily living _____
- ☐ Education   _____
- ☐ Work   _____
- ☐ Play   _____
- ☐ Leisure   _____
- ☐ Social participation   _____

2. Objects and their properties required:

3. Space demands:

4. Social demands:

5. Sequence and timing:

1.

2.

3.

4.

5.

6.

7.

8.

9.

10.

11.

12.

13.

14.

15.

6. Body functions required:

Function	How It Is Used	None	Minimally Challenged	Greatly Challenged
Judgment				
Concept formation				
Metacognition				
Cognitive flexibility				
Insight/awareness				
Sustained attention				
Selective attention				
Divided attention				
Short-term memory				
Working memory				
Long-term memory				
Discrimination of senses: Auditory				
Discrimination of senses: Tactile				
Discrimination of senses: Visual				
Discrimination of senses: Olfactory				
Discrimination of senses: Vestibular-proprioception				
Multisensory processing				
Sensory memory				
Spatial relationships				
Temporal relationships				
Recognition				
Categorization				
Generalization				
Awareness of reality				
Logical/coherent thought				
Appropriate thought content				
Execution of learned movements				
Coping				
Behavioral regulation				
Body image				
Self-concept				
Self-esteem				
Arousal				
Consciousness				
Orientation to self				
Orientation to place				
Orientation to time				
Orientation to others				
Emotional stability				
Motivation				
Impulse control				
Appetite				
Sleep				

Function	How It Is Used	None	Minimally Challenged	Greatly Challenged
Detection/registration				
Visual modulation				
Integration of senses				
Awareness at distances				
Tolerance of ambient sounds				
Location and distance of sounds				
Moving against gravity				
Taste				
Smell				
Body in space				
Comfort with touch				
Localizing pain				
Thermal awareness				
Joint range of motion				
Joint stability/alignment				
Strength				
Muscle tone				
Muscle endurance				
Stretch reflex				
ATNR				
STNR				
Righting and supporting reflex				
Eye–hand coordination				
Eye–foot coordination				
Bilateral coordination				
Crossing midline				
Fine motor control				
Gross motor control				
Oculomotor control				
Gait patterns				
Blood pressure				
Heart rate				
Respiratory rate				
Respiratory rhythm				
Respiratory depth				
Physical endurance, aerobic capacity				
Voice functions				
Voice rhythm and fluency				
Alternative vocalization				
Digestive system				
Metabolic system				
Endocrine system				

Function	How It Is Used	None	Minimally Challenged	Greatly Challenged
Urinary functions				
Genital and reproductive function				
Protective functions of the skin				
Repair functions of the skin				

7. Muscular analysis of movements required:

Muscle	Not Used	Minimally Challenged	Greatly Challenged
Shoulder flexion			
Shoulder extension			
Shoulder abduction			
Shoulder adduction			
Shoulder internal rotation			
Shoulder external rotation			
Elbow flexion			
Elbow extension			
Wrist supination			
Wrist pronation			
Wrist flexion			
Wrist extension			
Thumb flexion			
Thumb abduction			
Finger flexion			
Finger extension			
Trunk flexion			
Trunk extension			
Trunk rotation			
Lower extremities			

8. Performance skills required:

Skill	None	Low	High	How the Skill Is Used
Motor/praxis				
Sensory (perceptual)				
Emotional regulation				
Cognitive				
Communication/social				

Occupation-Based Activity Analysis Form

1. Occupation:

Area(s) of occupation: Subcategory:
- ☐ Activities of daily living   _____
- ☐ Instrumental activities of daily living _____
- ☐ Education   _____
- ☐ Work   _____
- ☐ Play   _____
- ☐ Leisure   _____
- ☐ Social Participation   _____

2. Values, beliefs, spirituality associated with participation:

3. Contexts:

Context	Supports	Inhibits
Physical/space demands		
Social		
Cultural		
Personal		
Temporal		
Virtual		

4. Objects and their properties used:

5. Social demands:

6. Sequence and timing:
   1.
   2.
   3.
   4.
   5.
   6.
   7.
   8.
   9.
   10.

7. Body functions required:

Function	Required?	How It Is Used
Judgment		
Concept formation		
Metacognition		
Cognitive flexibility		
Insight/awareness		
Sustained attention		
Selective attention		
Divided attention		
Short-term memory		
Working memory		
Long-term memory		
Discrimination of senses: Auditory		
Discrimination of senses: Tactile		
Discrimination of senses: Visual		
Discrimination of senses: Olfactory		
Discrimination of senses: Vestibular-proprioception		
Multisensory processing		
Sensory memory		
Spatial relationships		
Temporal relationships		
Recognition		
Categorization		
Generalization		
Awareness of reality		
Logical/coherent thought		
Appropriate thought content		
Execution of learned movements		
Coping		
Behavioral regulation		
Body image		
Self-concept		
Self-esteem		
Arousal		
Consciousness		
Orientation to self		
Orientation to place		
Orientation to time		
Orientation to others		
Emotional stability		
Motivation		
Impulse control		
Appetite		
Sleep		
Detection/registration		

Function	Required?	How It Is Used
Visual modulation		
Integration of senses		
Awareness at distances		
Tolerance of ambient sounds		
Location and distance of sounds		
Moving against gravity		
Taste		
Smell		
Body in space		
Comfort with touch		
Localizing pain		
Thermal awareness		
Joint range of motion		
Joint stability/alignment		
Strength		
Muscle tone		
Muscle endurance		
Stretch reflex		
ATNR		
STNR		
Righting and supporting reflex		
Eye–hand coordination		
Eye–foot coordination		
Bilateral coordination		
Crossing midline		
Fine motor control		
Gross motor control		
Oculomotor control		
Gait patterns		
Blood pressure		
Heart rate		
Respiratory rate		
Respiratory rhythm		
Respiratory depth		
Physical endurance, aerobic capacity		
Voice functions		
Voice rhythm and fluency		
Alternative vocalization		
Digestive system		
Metabolic system		
Endocrine system		
Urinary functions		
Genital and reproductive functions		
Protective functions of the skin		
Repair functions of the skin		

8. Muscular analysis of movements required:

Muscle	Required?
Shoulder flexion	
Shoulder extension	
Shoulder abduction	
Shoulder adduction	
Shoulder internal rotation	
Shoulder external rotation	
Elbow flexion	
Elbow extension	
Wrist supination	
Wrist pronation	
Wrist flexion	
Wrist extension	
Thumb flexion	
Thumb abduction	
Finger flexion	
Finger extension	
Trunk flexion	
Trunk extension	
Trunk rotation	
Lower extremities	

9. Performance skills required:

Skill	Required?	How the Skill Is Used
Motor/praxis		
Sensory (perceptual)		
Emotional regulation		
Cognitive		
Communication/social		

10. Performance patterns:

Parts of this occupation has elements of which of the following: (check all that apply)

✓	Pattern	Describe
	Useful habit	
	Dominating habit	
	Routine	
	Rituals	
	Roles	

COMPLETED
ACTIVITY ANALYSIS FORM

EXAMPLE OF A COMPLETED ACTIVITY ANALYSIS.

1. Occupation:

Area(s) of occupation for the client:	Subcategory:
☐ Activities of daily living	
☒ Instrumental activities of daily living	*Meal preparation*
☐ Education	
☐ Work	
☐ Play	
☐ Leisure	
☐ Social participation	

2. Objects and their properties:
   - *Tools: Nonstick frying pan, plastic spatula, bowl, fork, plate*
   - *Materials: Two fresh eggs, non-stick spray*
   - *Equipment: Trash can, stove*
     (Properties are listed with each item)

3. Space Demands:
   - *Adequate lighting to see the eggs in the pan*
   - *Space to stand and move in front of the stove*
   - *Flat counter to set eggs, bowl, and spatula on*

Thomas, H. *Occupation-Based Activity Analysis* (pp. 183-188). © 2012 SLACK Incorporated

4. Social demands:

- Clean up after cooking
- Eggs must be edible—not burned or undercooked
- Must have permission to use the stove or kitchen
- Wash hands before cooking
- Do not stick hands into the eggs

5. Sequence and timing:

1. Pick up the pan by grasping the handle of the pan with one hand and picking it up.
2. Grasp the can of non-stick spray with the other hand.
3. Hold the nozzle of the can over 6 inches above the pan.
4. Press the nozzle down and spray the entire surface of the pan quickly.
5. Set down the can of spray gently on the countertop.
6. Place the pan on top of the burner.
7. Turn on burner of stove by turning the burner knob to the right slowly until a clicking is heard.
8. Turn the knob to the left slowly until flame is at a medium level.
9. Grasp one egg with one hand.
10. Tap the egg against the edge of the counter until a crack is formed.
11. Bring the egg above the bowl quickly.
12. Using both hands, place thumbs into crack and pull shell apart gently, allowing egg to fall into bowl.
13. Place egg shell into trashcan.
14. Repeat steps 9 to 13 for the second egg
15. Hold the edge of the bowl with the left hand gently.
16. Pick up the fork along the flat edge using right hand.
17. Place fork into bowl and move fork in circular motion quickly.
18. Set fork down onto counter.
19. Pour eggs into pan carefully.
20. Grasp handle of pan with left hand, and pick up spatula with right hand. (Yes, I combined these two steps.)
21. Holding onto handle of pan, stir the eggs slowly with the tip of the spatula.
22. Continue to stir until eggs are fluffy and no longer watery.
23. Turn knob of stove to the off position until the flame goes out.
24. Pick up pan by grasping handle of pan and lifting up carefully.
25. Pick up the spatula along the handle.
26. Tilt pan over the plate and scrape eggs out of pan using the spatula.
27. Set down the pan on the burner.
28. Set down the spatula onto the counter top.

6. Body functions required:

Function	How it is used	None	Min	Great
Judgment	Need to decide when to put eggs in pan		X	
Concept formation		X		
Metacognition		X		
Cognitive flexibility	Use a different burner if one does not start		X	
Insight/awareness	Knowledge of one's ability and human ability		X	
Sustained attention	Must keep attention on cooking eggs or they will burn			X
Selective attention		X		
Divided attention		X		
Short-term memory	Recall what steps have been performed		X	
Working memory		X		
Long-term memory	Recall how scrambled eggs are made		X	
Discrimination of senses: Auditory	Hear popping, fire on stove		X	
Discrimination of senses: Tactile	Feel cracks in eggs as they are pulled apart		X	
Discrimination of senses: Visual	See where to put eggs; see consistency		X	
Discrimination of senses: Olfactory		X		
Discrimination of senses: Vestibular-proprioception	Proprioception in stirring eggs		X	
Multisensory processing	See and feel eggs as they cook		X	
Sensory memory	Consistency of eggs		X	
Spatial relationships	Pouring eggs into pan; reaching for spatula		X	
Temporal relationships	Time it takes to cook eggs		X	
Recognition	What the spatula is versus other objects		X	
Categorization		X		
Generalization		X		
Awareness of reality		X		
Logical/coherent thought		X		
Appropriate thought content		X		
Execution of learned movements	To crack eggs into bowl and stir eggs in pan			X
Coping		X		
Behavioral regulation		X		
Body image		X		
Self-concept		X		
Self-esteem		X		
Arousal	Must be alert to dangers			X
Consciousness	Must be conscious enough to avoid burning self			X
Orientation to self		X		
Orientation to place	Must know you are in a kitchen		X	
Orientation to time		X		
Orientation to others		X		
Emotional stability		X		
Motivation	Motivated to cook eggs from scratch		X	
Impulse control		X		

Function	How it is used	None	Min	Great
Appetite		X		
Sleep		X		
Detection/registration	See all objects in environment		X	
Visual modulation	Focus on eggs in pan		X	
Integration of senses	See and feel eggs as they are stirred		X	
Awareness at distances	Up from eggs and then back down		X	
Tolerance of ambient sounds		X		
Location and distance of sounds		X		
Moving against gravity	Standing upright, arms away from body		X	
Taste		X		
Smell		X		
Body in space		X		
Comfort with touch	Touching eggs and shells as they are pulled apart		X	
Localizing pain		X		
Thermal awareness	As hands are near pan		X	
Joint range of motion	To reach eggs, pan, hold spatula and to stir.		X	
Joint stability/alignment		X		
Strength	To break eggs apart and to stir		X	
Muscle tone	To hold eggs without dropping		X	
Muscle endurance	Standing at stove; stirring		X	
Stretch reflex		X		
ATNR		X		
STNR		X		
Righting and supporting reflex		X		
Eye–hand coordination	Reaching for spatula; cracking eggs over bowl		X	
Eye–foot coordination		X		
Bilateral coordination	Cracking eggs, holding pan and stirring			X
Crossing midline		X		
Fine motor control	Cracking eggs; opening egg container		X	
Gross motor control	Stirring; picking up pan or bowl		X	
Oculomotor control	Binocularity to reach for objects		X	
Gait patterns		X		
Blood pressure		X		
Heart rate		X		
Respiratory rate		X		
Respiratory rhythm		X		
Respiratory depth		X		
Physical endurance, aerobic capacity	Standing and stirring		X	
Voice functions		X		
Voice rhythm and fluency		X		
Alternative vocalization		X		
Digestive system		X		
Metabolic system		X		
Endocrine system		X		

Function	How it is used	None	Min	Great
Urinary functions		X		
Genital and reproductive functions		X		
Protective functions of the skin	*Cracking eggs (shells are sharp)*		X	
Repair functions of the skin		X		

7. Muscular analysis of movements required:

Muscle	Not used	Min	Great
Shoulder flexion		X	
Shoulder extension		X	
Shoulder abduction		X	
Shoulder adduction		X	
Shoulder internal rotation		X	
Shoulder external rotation		X	
Elbow flexion		X	
Elbow extension		X	
Wrist supination		X	
Wrist pronation		X	
Wrist flexion		X	
Wrist extension		X	
Thumb flexion		X	
Thumb abduction	X		
Finger flexion		X	
Finger extension		X	
Trunk flexion	X		
Trunk extension	X		
Trunk rotation		X	
Lower extremities		X	

8. Performance skills required:

Skill	None	Low	High	Examples of how the skill is used
Motor/praxis		X		*Stirring; picking up objects; cracking eggs*
Sensory (perceptual)		X		*Seeing where the eggs are; feeling the consistency of eggs as they cook*
Emotional regulation	X			
Cognitive		X		*Deciding when the eggs are cooked*
Communication/social	X			

INDEX

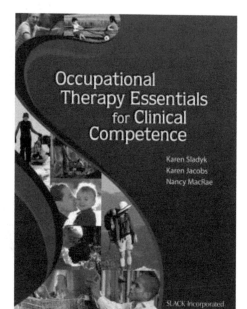

Attention Industry Partners!

Whether you are interested in buying multiple copies of a book, chapter reprints, or looking for something new and different — we are able to accommodate your needs.

MULTIPLE COPIES

At attractive discounts starting for purchases as low as 25 copies for a single title, SLACK Incorporated will be able to meet all of your needs.

CHAPTER REPRINTS

SLACK Incorporated is able to offer the chapters you want in a format that will lead to success. Bound with an attractive cover, use the chapters that are a fit specifically for your company. Available for quantities of 100 or more.

CUSTOMIZE

SLACK Incorporated is able to create a specialized custom version of any of our products specifically for your company.

Please contact the Marketing Communications Director for further details on multiple copy purchases, chapter reprints or custom printing at 1-800-257-8290 or 1-856-848-1000.

*Please note all conditions are subject to change.

SLACK®
INCORPORATED
Health Care Books and Journals • 6900 Grove Road • Thorofare, NJ 08086

1-800-257-8290
Fax: 1-856-848-6091
E-mail: orders@slackinc.com

www.slackbooks.com

CODE: 328